A YEAR
of Easy
KETO
Desserts

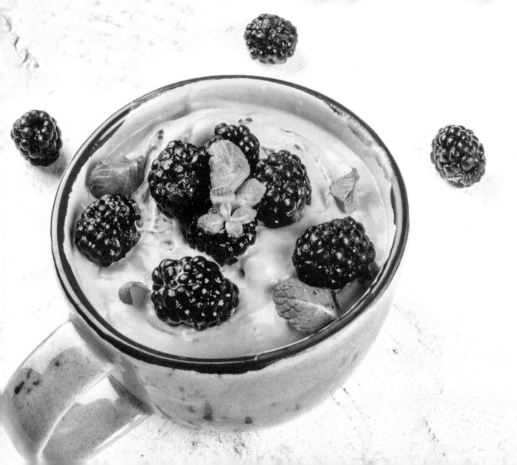

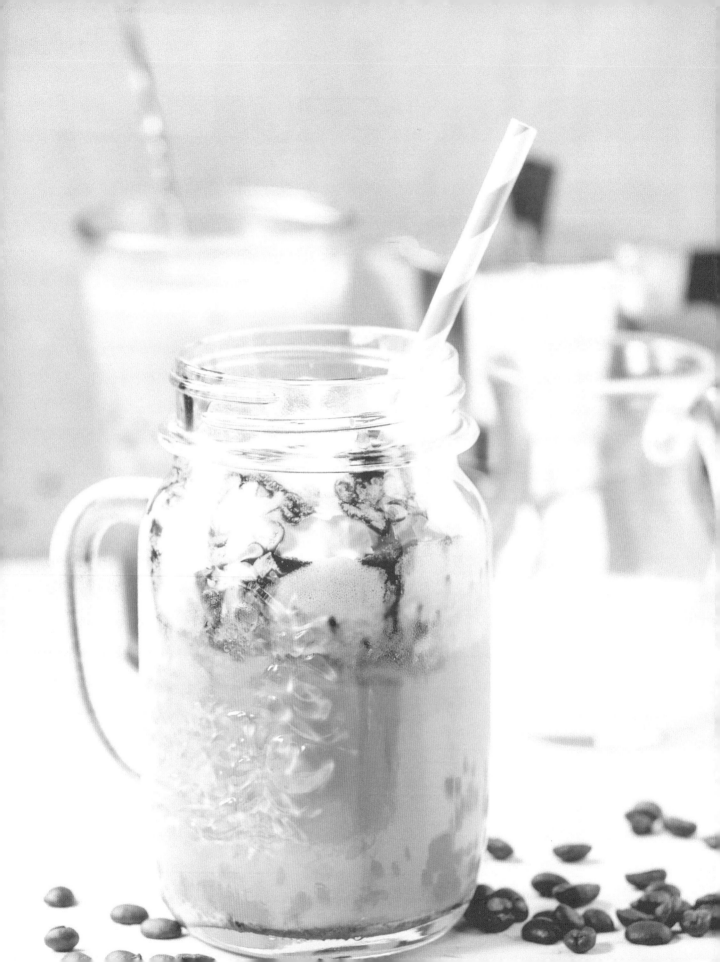

INTRODUCTION

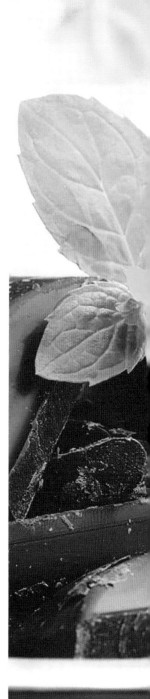

F ollowing a ketogenic diet can often feel like the fun is taken out of eating a favorite sweet treat. In fact, a ketogenic diet doesn't even allow for our favorite treats anymore which is why I was inspired to write this book.

I wanted to create a cookbook that was full of delicious and easy to make keto-friendly desserts that weren't going to knock you out of ketosis. I wanted to create dessert options that you can enjoy without feeling like you are taking a "cheat day."

In this book, you will find recipes for all four seasons from fall to winter, to the warmer spring and summer months. And, the best part is that each recipe will only cost you five grams of net carbs or less!

I hope this dessert book becomes a staple in your kitchen and that it brings a little joy back into creating and enjoying some guilt-free treats.

I would love to hear any feedback from you, and if you have any questions regarding any of the recipes at all, please do not hesitate to email me at:

Elizabeth@ketojane.com

You may also like

HOMEMADE KETO SOUP

http://ketojane.com/soup

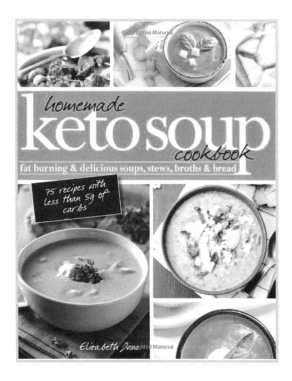

The answer to your keto dinnertime dilemma. Easy keto and low-carb friendly soups and stews to satisfy your soul, all with *less than 5g of net carbs!*

KETO BREAD BAKERS COOKBOOK

http://ketojane.com/bread

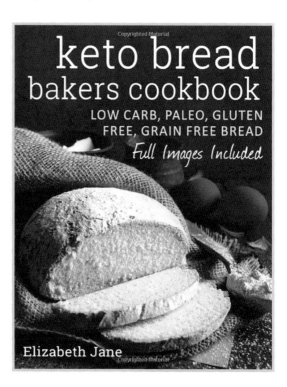

Everyone loves bread! And if you're on a special diet and miss bread, then this book is for you! Paleo, low carb, gluten free, keto, wheat free, but still the same great tastes.

The Keto Bread Makers cookbook contains all the bread that you thought you had to give up.

Free Easy Keto Meals

I am delighted you have chosen my book to help you start or continue on your keto journey.

Keto meals can be hard, complicated ingredients, long cooking times… to help you stay on the keto track, I am pleased to offer you three mini ebooks from my 'Keto Easy Meals Bonus Series', completely free of charge! These three mini ebooks cover how to make everything from easy breakfasts, to 6 ingredient dinners and meals using just one pot (less prep and washing up)!

Simply visit the link below to get your free copy of all three mini ebooks:

http://ketojane.com/ketomeals

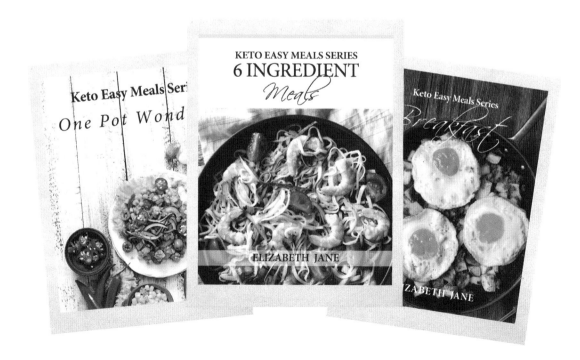

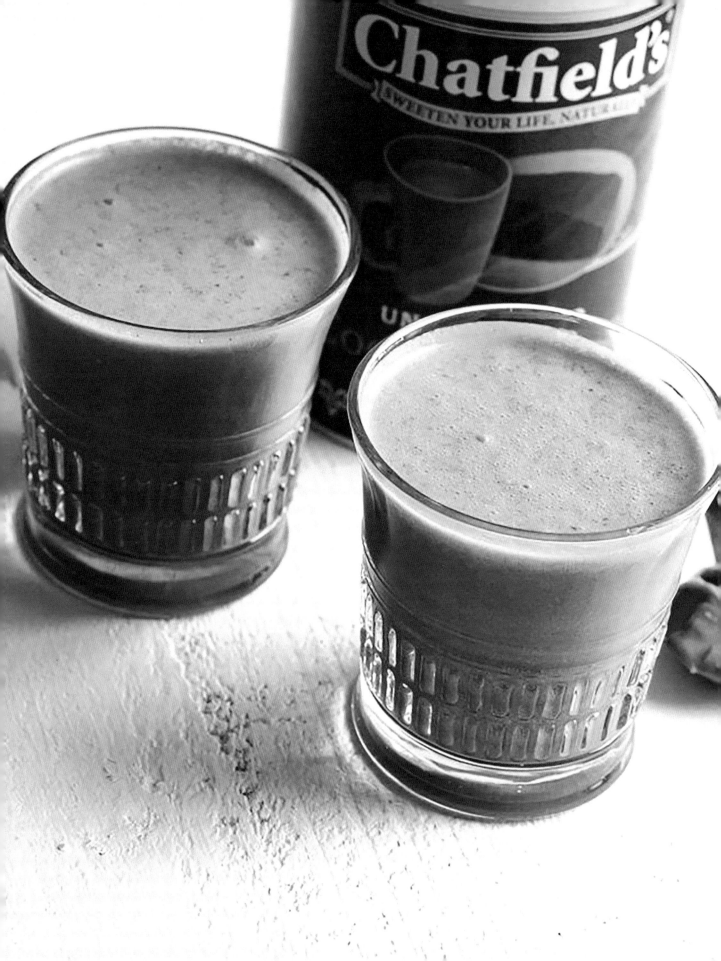

CONTENTS

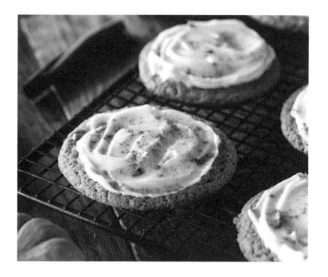

Fall Recipes 17

COOKIES 18

FUDGE/SAVORY BITES 21

DONUTS/SCONES 25

DESSERT BEVERAGES 27

COLD TREATS 28

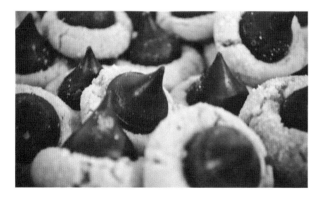

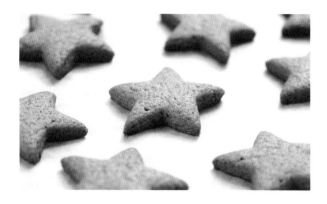

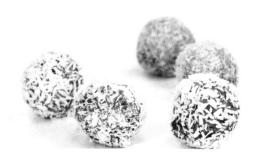

Summer Recipes 61

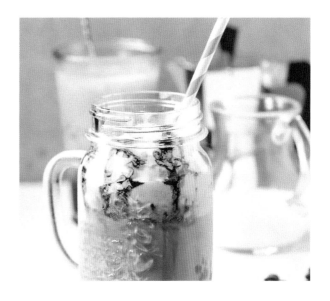

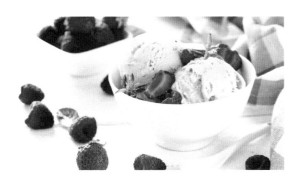

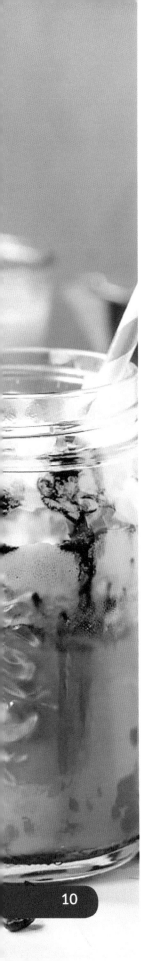

HOW THIS
Book Works

This cookbook contains helpful baking tips to help you get the best results possible. There are also serving suggestions included to give you an idea about what each of these recipes pair well with.

You will also notice there are five symbols on the top right-hand side of each recipe. A key to these symbols is set out below:

PREPARATION TIME:

Time required to prepare the recipe. This does not include cooking time.

COOKING TIME:

Time required to cook the recipe. This does not include the preparation time.

SERVINGS:

How many servings each recipe requires. This can be adjusted. For example, by doubling the quantity of all of the ingredients, you can make twice as many servings.

DIFFICULTY LEVEL:

1 An easy-to-make recipe that can be put together with a handful of ingredients and in a short amount of time.

2 These recipes are a little more difficult and time-consuming but are still easy enough, even for beginners!

3 A more advanced recipe for the adventurous baker. You will not see too many Level 3 recipes in this book. These recipes are ideal for when you have a little bit more time to spare.

COST:

$: A low-budget everyday dessert recipe.

$$: A moderately priced, middle-of-the-road dessert recipe.

$$$: A more expensive recipe that is great for serving at a party. These recipes contain higher-priced ingredients.

DIETARY LABELS

I have also included dietary labels for each recipe so you can quickly see if a recipe is vegetarian, gluten-free, dairy-free, or Paleo.

 Gluten-free

 Dairy-free

 Vegetarian

 Paleo

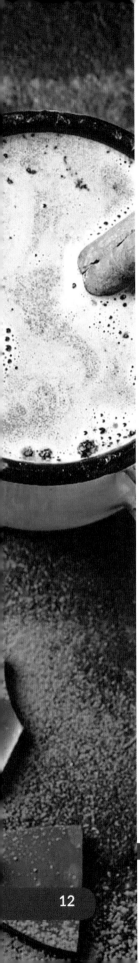

YOUR GUIDE TO MAKING DELICIOUS
Keto Desserts

To help you get started, I put together a quick guide on how you can get the most out of baking and how you can make whipping up keto desserts fun and delicious.

Here are some tips to help you make the most delicious keto dessert you've tried yet!

#1   **FOCUS ON QUALITY:** Quality is really going to matter here. I made sure to keep these recipes simple enough where you can actually taste that vanilla extract or taste the hints of shredded coconut. You want to be able to taste these flavors, so focus on a getting a high-quality pure vanilla extract and high-quality baking spices to really bring the flavors out.

 # 2   **GET THE NATURALLY FLAVORED STEVIA:** You will find I use stevia in many of these recipes for a couple of reasons. For one, it keeps the carb count down, and number two, you can get some flavored stevia options (my personal favorite is the vanilla cream) that adds a nice touch to your baking recipes. Just be sure to stick to the ones that are naturally flavored VS artificial.

 # 3   **FOCUS ON THE FAT:** Us keto-dieters are used to adding lots of fat into our diet, and when it comes to these dessert recipes, I have used a lot of coconut oil and butter, so be sure to stock up on these! You will be using them liberally in many of the recipes.

 # 4   **MAKE IT PALEO:** Looking to make your recipes Paleo-friendly? Try swapping out the dairy by using coconut milk instead of milk and coconut oil instead of butter.

 # 5   **HAVE FUN:** Not everyone loves to bake, so I tried to make these recipes simple and not very time-consuming so we could bring some fun back to baking keto-friendly desserts. Have fun with it! After all, the end result will be a delicious treat you can enjoy without the guilt.

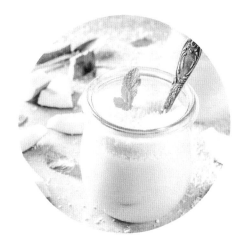

USEFUL KITCHEN EQUIPMENT FOR KETO
Dessert Baking

Below are my recommended 'tools' for making amazing desserts. If you do not have them yet, I have linked to my recommended purchases (which I personally use!) on Amazon.

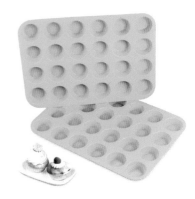

- Silicone mini cupcake pan
- Non-stick silicone baking spatulas
- 9X13 baking pan
- Unbleached parchment paper
- Silicone Whisk Set

- Sugar-Free Chocolate Syrup
- Natural Food Coloring
- Liquid Vanilla Cream Stevia
- Popsicle Mold Set
- Vitamix Blender
- Silicone Baking Mat
- Cookie cooling rack
- My favorite stainless steel measuring spoons
- Stackable measuring cups
- Glass storage containers

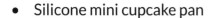

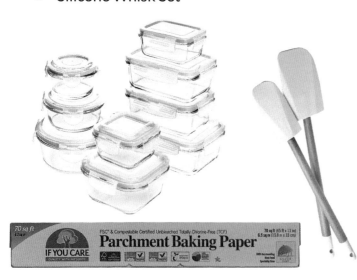

KETO BAKING STAPLE INGREDIENT
Shopping List

*H*ere is a list of some of the staple ingredients you will be needing for many of the recipes found in this book.

SWEETENERS

Stevia

Swerve

Monk fruit

FATS/OILS

Coconut oil

Full-fat canned coconut milk

FLOUR

Almond flour

DAIRY & EGGS

Butter

Eggs

OTHER BAKING NECESSITIES

Pure vanilla extract

Baking powder

Ground cinnamon

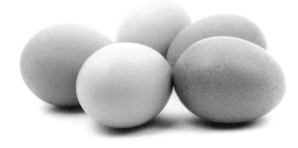

A NOTE ON SWEETENERS &
Specialty Ingredients

*A*s a way to add variation to these dessert recipes, you will find a variety of low-carb sweeteners used. However, feel free to swap one for the other. For example, if you prefer stevia over erythritol, use stevia! If you can't find monk fruit, you can try using Swerve instead. Feel free to be creative, and use whatever low-carb sweetener you prefer in each recipe.

The same goes for certain specialty ingredients like aluminum-free baking powder. For the purpose of making many of these recipes Paleo friendly in addition to keto-approved, you will find that a recipe calls for aluminum and gluten-free baking powder. Feel free to use regular baking powder if you are unable to find the aluminum and gluten-free version.

Many recipes also call for liquid vanilla stevia, but you can feel free to use regular liquid stevia, or a flavor of your choice!

You will also come across some recipes that call for ghee. If you are unable to find ghee, feel free to use butter instead.

These recipes are designed to be delicious and bring the fun back into baking keto desserts, so feel free to adjust the ingredients to your taste and preference!

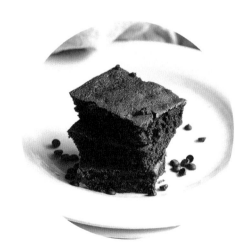

FALL *Recipes*

COOKIES

Peanut Butter Thumbprint Cookies

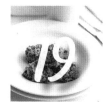

The Ultimate Fall Spice Keto Chocolate Chip Cookies

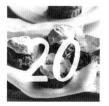

Nutmeg & Cinnamon Cookies With No-Carb Vanilla Icing

FUDGE/SAVORY BITES

Pumpkin Cheesecake Fat Bombs
21

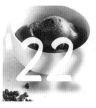

Sea Salt & Caramel Fudge Savory Bites

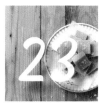

Peanut Butter Fudge

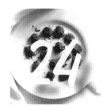

Chocolate Truffles

DONUTS/SCONE

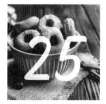

Cinnamon & Clove Donuts

Maple Cinnamon Scones
26

DESSERT BEVERAGES

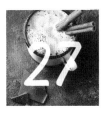

Fall Spiced Hot Chocolate

COLD TREATS

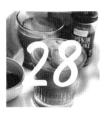

Pumpkin-Spiced Cacao Mousse

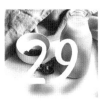

Coconut Cream Pumpkin Pie Milkshake

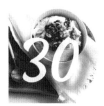

Maple Walnut Whipped Cream

PEANUT BUTTER THUMBPRINT *Cookies*

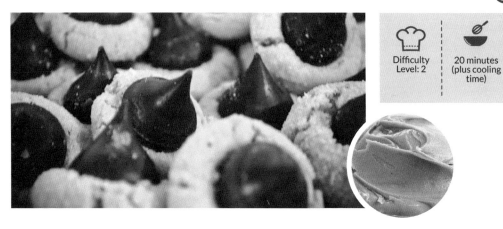

Difficulty Level: 2	20 minutes (plus cooling time)	8-10 minutes	x16 (1 cookie per serving) $$

GF DF

INGREDIENTS:

- 2 cups unsweetened peanut butter (use almond butter for a paleo version)
- 2 eggs
- 2 tsp. liquid stevia
- 1 tsp. pure vanilla extract
- 1 tsp. gluten- and aluminum-free baking powder

Filling:

- ½ cup coconut oil
- ½ cup of dark unsweetened chocolate chips

Nutritional Information:	
Carbs: 8g	**Fat:** 27g
Fiber: 3g	**Protein:** 8g
Net Carbs: 5g	**Calories:** 298

DIRECTIONS:

1. Preheat the oven to 350 degrees F and line a baking sheet with parchment paper.
2. Add the peanut butter and eggs to a mixing bowl and stir.
3. Add in the remaining ingredients and mix well.
4. Drop by 1-inch rounds onto the parchment-lined baking sheet.
5. Using your thumb, press into the center of each cookie.
6. Bake for 8-10 minutes or until the edges begin to brown.
7. While the cookies are baking, add the coconut oil and dark chocolate chips to a stockpot over low to medium heat and stir until melted.
8. Once the cookies are done, scoop about 1 teaspoon of the chocolate mixture into the center of each cookie.
9. Allow the chocolate center to harden and enjoy.

Preparation Instructions:

You can also use sugar-free jam in the center of these cookies if you aren't a fan of chocolate. Add the jam before the cookies go into the oven.

Serving Suggestions:

Serve with a glass of unsweetened almond milk.

THE ULTIMATE FALL SPICE KETO CHOCOLATE CHIP *Cookies*

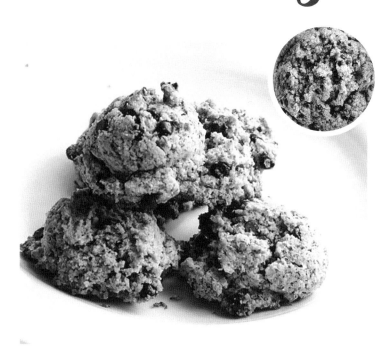

Difficulty Level: 2	10 minutes (plus cooling time)	14-16 minutes	x12 (1 cookie per serving) $$

GF

INGREDIENTS:

- 2 cups finely ground almond flour
- 2 eggs
- ½ cup butter, melted (use coconut oil for a paleo version)
- ½ cup raw cacao nibs
- 3 Tbsp. monk fruit sweetener
- 1 tsp. gluten- and aluminum-free baking powder
- 1 tsp. pumpkin pie spice
- ½ tsp. ground cinnamon
- 1 tsp. pure vanilla extract
- ½ tsp. sea salt

DIRECTIONS:

1. Preheat the oven to 350 degrees F and line a baking sheet with parchment paper.
2. Add the melted butter, vanilla, and eggs to a mixing bowl and whisk.
3. Add all of the dry ingredients to a mixing bowl minus the cacao nibs and mix well.
4. Whisk the wet mixture into the dry and whisk until no lumps remain.
5. Fold in the cacao nibs.
6. Drop by the rounded tablespoon, making 12 large cookies onto the parchment-lined baking sheet and bake for 14-16 minutes or until the edges begin to brown.
7. Cool and enjoy!

Preparation Instructions:

You can also use unsweetened dark chocolate chips if you are unable to find raw cacao nibs.

Serving Suggestions:

Serve with a glass of unsweetened almond milk.

Nutritional Information:

Carbs: 6g

Fiber: 2g

Net Carbs: 4g

Fat: 14g

Protein: 3g

Calories: 158

NUTMEG & CINNAMON *Cookies*

WITH NO-CARB VANILLA ICING

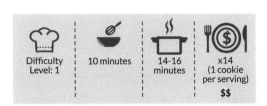

Difficulty Level: 1 | 10 minutes | 14-16 minutes | x14 (1 cookie per serving) $$

GF

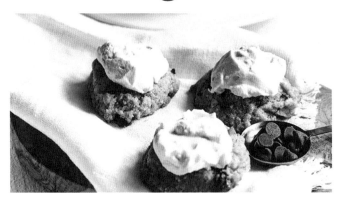

INGREDIENTS:

- 2 ½ cups finely ground almond flour
- 2 eggs
- ½ cup butter, melted (use coconut oil for a paleo version)
- 3 Tbsp. monk fruit sweetener (use pure maple syrup for a paleo version)
- 1 tsp. gluten- and aluminum-free baking powder
- 1 tsp. ground nutmeg
- 1 tsp. ground cinnamon
- 1 tsp. pure vanilla extract
- ½ tsp. sea salt

Frosting:

- 1 cup heavy whipping cream (use unsweetened coconut cream for a paleo version)
- ¼ cup Swerve (use pure maple syrup for a paleo version)
- 2 tsp. pure vanilla extract

Nutritional Information:	
Carbs: 6g	**Fat:** 13g
Fiber: 1g	**Protein:** 2g
Net Carbs: 5g	**Calories:** 130

DIRECTIONS:

1. Preheat the oven to 350 degrees F and line a baking sheet with parchment paper.
2. Add the melted butter, vanilla and eggs to a mixing bowl and whisk.
3. Add all dry ingredients except cacao nibs to a mixing bowl and mix well.
4. Whisk the wet mixture into the dry and whisk until no lumps remain.
5. Drop by the rounded tablespoon, making 14 cookies onto the parchment-lined baking sheet and bake for 14-16 minutes or until the edges begin to brown.
6. While the cookies are baking, make the vanilla frosting by adding all ingredients to a high-speed blender, or add to a mixing bowl and, using a hand mixer, whip until soft peaks form.
7. Allow the cookies to cool, and then top with a dollop of the vanilla frosting.

Preparation Instructions:

You can add a tablespoon of raw, unsweetened cocoa to make these cookies even more decadent.

Serving Suggestions:

Serve with a glass of unsweetened almond milk.

PUMPKIN CHEESECAKE
Fat Bombs

INGREDIENTS:

- 1 cup whipped cream cheese
- 2 Tbsp. ghee
- ¼ cup pure pumpkin puree
- 1 tsp. pumpkin pie spice
- 1 tsp. pure vanilla extract
- 10 drops liquid vanilla stevia

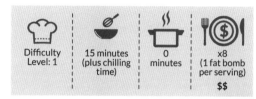

Difficulty Level: 1 | 15 minutes (plus chilling time) | 0 minutes | x8 (1 fat bomb per serving) $$

DIRECTIONS:

1. Add the whipped cream cheese, ghee, and pumpkin puree to a food processor or blender and blend until the mixture is mixed and "fluffy."
2. Add the pumpkin pie spice, vanilla extract, and stevia and whip again.
3. Pour the mixture into silicone baking molds. Alternatively, line mini muffin tins with muffin liners, and scoop about 1 tablespoon of the mixture into each mold or muffin liner.
4. Freeze for about 1 hour before serving, and store leftovers in the freezer.

Preparation Instructions:

You can use regular butter instead of ghee if preferred.

Serving Suggestions:

Serve with a mug of hot coffee or tea for a delicious after-dinner treat.

Nutritional Information:

Carbs: 5g

Fiber: 0g

Net Carbs: 5g

Fat: 13g

Protein: 2g

Calories: 133

SEA SALT & CARAMEL FUDGE SAVORY *Bites*

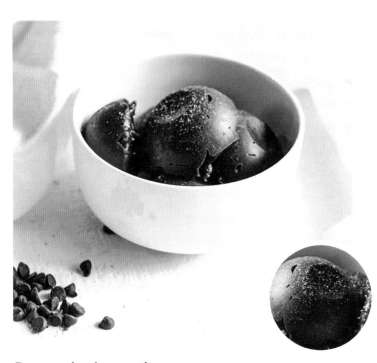

Difficulty Level: 1	15 minutes (plus chilling time)	0 minutes	x10 (1 bite per serving) $$

GF DF V

INGREDIENTS:

- 1 cup coconut oil
- 10 drops vanilla liquid stevia
- ¼ cup raw unsweetened cocoa powder
- 1 tsp. pure vanilla extract
- 1 tsp. sugar-free caramel extract
- 1 pinch sea salt

DIRECTIONS:

1. Line mini cupcake tins with cupcake liners and add the coconut oil and stevia to a mixing bowl and whip with a handheld mixer.
2. Add the cocoa powder, vanilla, caramel extract, and salt.
3. Pour into the lined muffin tins and freeze for about 20 minutes or until set.
4. Enjoy and store leftovers covered in the freezer.

Preparation Instructions:

You can also use silicone cupcake molds to make these.

Serving Suggestions:

Serve with a glass of unsweetened almond milk.

Nutritional Information:	
Carbs: 1g	**Fat:** 22g
Fiber: 1g	**Protein:** 0g
Net Carbs: 0g	**Calories:** 194

PEANUT BUTTER *Fudge*

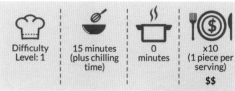

Difficulty Level: 1 | 15 minutes (plus chilling time) | 0 minutes | x10 (1 piece per serving) $$

GF | DF | V

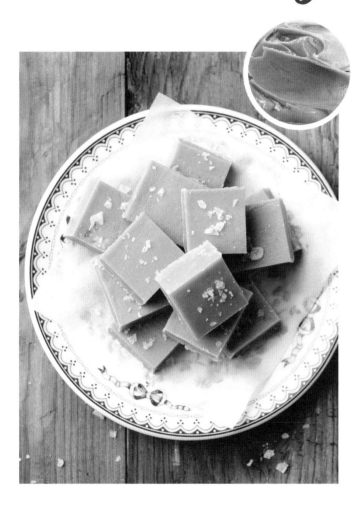

INGREDIENTS:

- 1 cup coconut oil
- 10 drops liquid stevia
- ½ cup unsweetened peanut butter (use almond butter for a paleo version)
- 1 tsp. pure vanilla extract
- 1 pinch sea salt

DIRECTIONS:

1. Line a baking sheet with parchment paper and add the coconut oil and stevia to a mixing bowl and whip with a handheld mixer.
2. Add the peanut butter, vanilla, and salt.
3. Scoop the mixture onto the lined baking sheet and flatten to about 1-inch thick.
4. Freeze for about 20 minutes or until set and cut into small squares.
5. Store leftovers covered in the freezer.

Nutritional Information:

Carbs: 3g	**Fat:** 28g
Fiber: 1g	**Protein:** 2g
Net Carbs: 2g	**Calories:** 261

Preparation Instructions:

You can also make these into mini fudge bites using mini cupcake silicone molds.

Serving Suggestions:

Serve with a cup of tea or coffee.

CHOCOLATE
Truffles

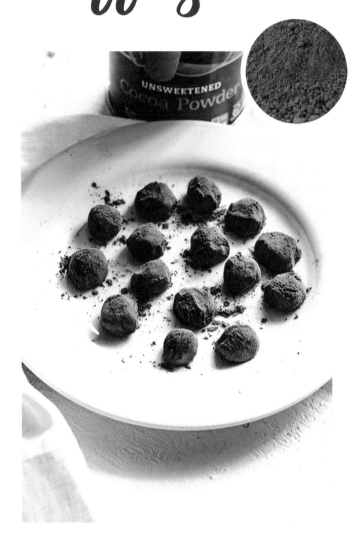

Difficulty Level: 2	10 minutes (plus chilling time)	5 minutes	18 (1 truffle per serving) $$

GF

INGREDIENTS:

- 1 cup unsweetened dark chocolate chips
- 4 Tbsp. butter
- ¾ cup heavy cream
- ¼ cup Swerve
- ½ tsp. pure vanilla extract
- ½ cup raw unsweetened cocoa powder for coating

DIRECTIONS:

1. Add the chocolate chips and butter to a stockpot over low heat. Stir until melted.
2. Mix in the Swerve and vanilla extract.
3. Remove from heat and stir in the heavy cream.
4. Refrigerate the mixture for at least 4 hours.
5. Once chilled, scoop the hardened chocolate mixture out with a small cookie scoop and drop onto a parchment-lined baking sheet.
6. Sprinkle with the cocoa powder and refrigerate until ready to enjoy.

Nutritional Information:

Carbs: 8g	**Fat:** 12g
Fiber: 3g	**Protein:** 2g
Net Carbs: 5g	**Calories:** 135

Preparation Instructions:

You can use 1 teaspoon of stevia in place of Swerve if desired.

Serving Suggestions:

Serve with a cup of tea or coffee.

CINNAMON & CLOVE *Donuts*

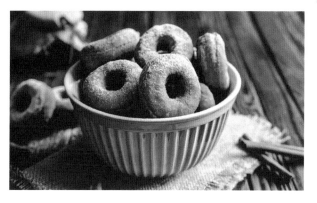

Difficulty Level: 2	20 minutes	0 minutes	x6 (1 donut per serving) $$

GF

INGREDIENTS:

- 1 cup finely ground almond flour
- 2 eggs
- ¼ cup unsalted butter, melted (use melted ghee for a paleo version)
- ¼ cup heavy cream (use full-fat unsweetened coconut milk for a paleo version)
- 1 tsp. ground cinnamon
- ¼ tsp. ground cloves
- 2 tsp. aluminum and gluten-free baking powder
- 1 tsp. pure vanilla extract
- 2 tsp. liquid stevia
- Coconut oil for greasing

Cinnamon & Clove Coating:

- ½ cup melted coconut oil
- 2 Tbsp. monk fruit in the raw sweetener
- 1 Tbsp. ground cinnamon
- ¼ tsp. ground cloves

Nutritional Information:

Carbs: 4g	**Fat:** 31g
Fiber: 2g	**Protein:** 3g
Net Carbs: 2g	**Calories:** 299

DIRECTIONS:

1. Preheat the oven to 350 degrees F and grease a donut pan
2. Make the donut mixture by adding all the dry ingredients to a large mixing bowl and stir.
3. Whisk the eggs, melted butter, heavy cream, vanilla, and stevia in a separate bowl, and then whisk slowly into the dry mixture. Whisk until no lumps remain.
4. Pour the mixture into the pregreased donut pan and bake for 20-25 minutes.
5. While the donuts are baking, make the cinnamon and clove coating by whisking together monk fruit, cinnamon, and ground cloves in a large mixing bowl. Set aside.
6. Once the donuts are done, allow them to cool and then melt the coconut oil in a large mixing bowl. Dunk each donut into the melted oil, covering both sides.
7. Immediately sprinkle with the cinnamon and clove mixture. Also sprinkle on some powdered stevia if desired.

Preparation Instructions:

If you aren't a fan of cloves, you can use cinnamon, increasing the amount to 1¼ teaspoon in the donut mixture and 1¼ tablespoon in the coating mixture.

Serving Suggestions:

Serve with a dollop of cream cheese if desired.

MAPLE CINNAMON *Scones*

INGREDIENTS:

- 1¼ cups finely ground almond flour
- ¼ cup unsweetened coconut milk
- 1 egg
- ¼ cup monk fruit sweetener
- 1 tsp. gluten- and aluminum-free baking powder
- 2 Tbsp. butter, melted (use melted coconut oil for a paleo option)
- 1 tsp. pure vanilla extract
- 1 tsp. ground cinnamon
- 1 tsp. sugar-free maple extract (use 1 Tbsp. pure maple syrup for a paleo version)
- ½ tsp. sea salt

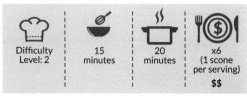

Difficulty Level: 2 | 15 minutes | 20 minutes | x6 (1 scone per serving) $$

GF

DIRECTIONS:

1. Preheat the oven to 350 degrees F and line a baking sheet with parchment paper.
2. Add the dry ingredients to a large mixing bowl and mix well.
3. Add the coconut milk, the egg, melted butter, vanilla extract, and maple extract. Mix well.
4. Form the dough into a large round and place on the baking sheet and flatten to about 1-inch thick.
5. Cut into 6 wedges and bake for about 20 minutes or until the edges begin to brown.
6. Cool and enjoy!

Preparation Instructions:

You can add fresh fruit like raspberries to the batter if desired.

Serving Suggestions:

Serve with whipped cream cheese if desired.

Nutritional Information:
Carbs: 3g
Fiber: 2g
Net Carbs: 1g
Fat: 10g
Protein: 3g
Calories: 105

SPICED HOT
Chocolate

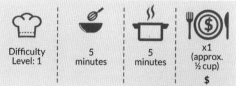

Difficulty Level: 1	5 minutes	5 minutes	x1 (approx. ½ cup) $

GF DF V

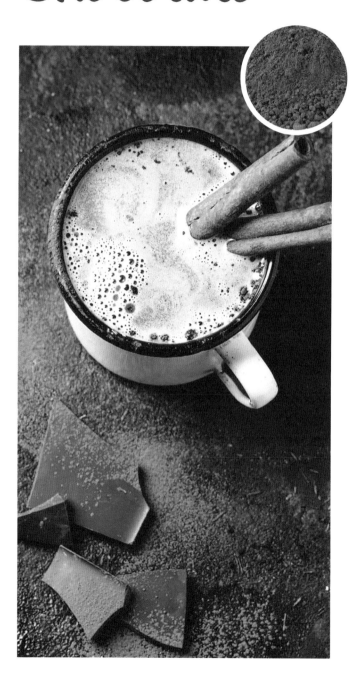

INGREDIENTS:

- ½ cup full-fat unsweetened coconut milk
- 1 Tbsp. raw unsweetened cocoa powder
- ¼ tsp. ground cinnamon
- ⅛ tsp. ground nutmeg
- ⅛ tsp. ground cloves
- 1 tsp. pure. Vanilla extract
- 1 drop vanilla cream liquid stevia

DIRECTIONS:

1. Add all the ingredients to a stockpot over low or medium heat and whisk until warmed through.
2. Pour into your favorite mug and enjoy!

Preparation Instructions:

Add a pinch of pumpkin spice if desired.

Serving Suggestions:

Serve with a dollop of unsweetened whipped cream if desired.

Nutritional Information:	
Carbs: 10g	**Fat:** 30g
Fiber: 5g	**Protein:** 4g
Net Carbs: 5g	**Calories:** 292

Cold Treats
PUMPKIN-SPICED CACAO *Mousse*

Difficulty Level: 1	15 minutes (plus chilling time)	0 minutes	x4 (approx. ¼ cup per serving) $$

GF DF V P

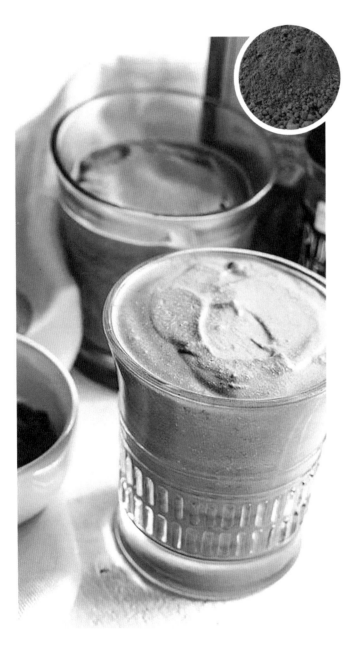

INGREDIENTS:

- 2 cups of canned unsweetened full-fat coconut milk (place can in the refrigerator overnight)
- ½ cup pure pumpkin puree
- 2 Tbsp. raw unsweetened cacao powder
- ½ tsp. pumpkin pie spice
- 10 drops liquid vanilla stevia

DIRECTIONS:

1. Add the coconut cream to a blender or food processor, and whip for about 2 minutes until creamy.
2. Add remaining ingredients and blend until combined.
3. Scoop the mixture into 4 small serving glasses or bowls, and chill for at least 1 hour before serving.

Serving Suggestions:

Serve with an extra sprinkle of pumpkin pie spice if desired.

Nutritional Information:	
Carbs: 5g	**Fat:** 8g
Fiber: 2g	**Protein:** 1g
Net Carbs: 3g	**Calories:** 87

COCONUT CREAM
PUMPKIN *Pie Milkshake*

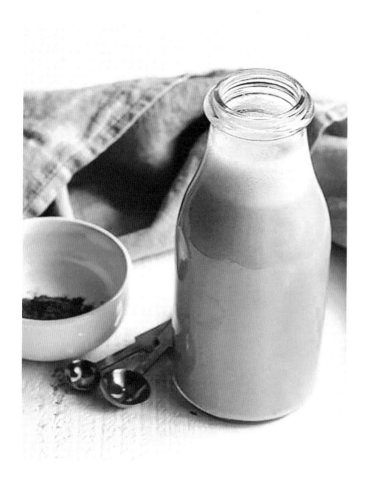

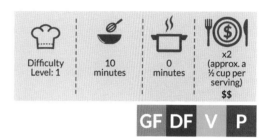

Difficulty Level: 1 | 10 minutes | 0 minutes | x2 (approx. a ½ cup per serving) $$

GF DF V P

DIRECTIONS:

1. Add all ingredients to a high-speed blender and blend until smooth.
2. Enjoy right away.

Preparation Instructions:

For canned coconut milk, blend the contents of the can first to combine the coconut milk and cream evenly.

Serving Suggestions:

If you are not avoiding dairy, you can also make this recipe using heavy cream.

INGREDIENTS:

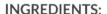

- 1 cup full-fat unsweetened coconut milk
- ¼ cup pure pumpkin puree
- ¼ tsp. pumpkin pie spice
- 1 tsp. pure vanilla extract

Nutritional Information:

Carbs: 8g   **Fat:** 29g

Fiber: 3g   **Protein:** 3g

Net Carbs: 5g **Calories:** 288

MAPLE WALNUT
Whipped Cream

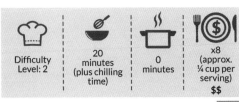

Difficulty Level: 2 | 20 minutes (plus chilling time) | 0 minutes | x8 (approx. ¼ cup per serving) $$

GF

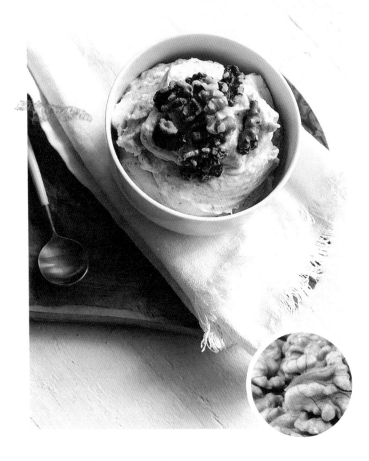

INGREDIENTS:

- 2 cups heavy whipping cream
- 2 Tbsp. ghee
- 2 tsp. sugar-free maple extract
- 1 tsp. pure vanilla extract
- 1 cup chopped walnuts
- 10 drops liquid vanilla stevia
- ½ tsp. guar gum

DIRECTIONS:

1. Place a large mixing bowl in the fridge to chill for about 20 minutes.
2. Remove the chilled bowl and add the heavy whipping cream. Whip using a handheld blender until stiff peaks form.
3. Add the remaining ingredients minus the walnuts and guar gum. Whip until combined.
4. Fold the chopped walnuts and guar gum in gently and store in an airtight container in the freezer overnight or for at least 8 hours before enjoying.

Preparation Instructions:

You can make this ahead of time, store in the fridge, and then whip one more time before serving.

Serving Suggestions:

Serve with a bowl of your favorite keto ice cream.

Nutritional Information:

Carbs: 3g	**Fat:** 24g
Fiber: 1g	**Protein:** 4g
Net Carbs: 2g	**Calories:** 230

COOKIES

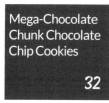

Mega-Chocolate Chunk Chocolate Chip Cookies

32

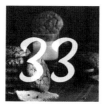

33

Chewy Brownie Mini Cookies

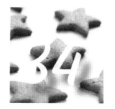

34

Keto Gingerbread Cookies

Snowflake Christmas Spice Sugar Cookies

35

SAVORY BITES & CHOCOLATE

The Ultimate Low-Carb Apple Pie Savory Bites

36

Valentine's Day Chocolate Raspberry Fat Bombs

37

Dark Chocolate Peppermint Bark

38

BROWNIES, PIES & LOAF BREAD

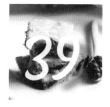

39

Blondies

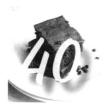

40

Eggnog Brownies

Christmas-Inspired Pecan Pie Savory Bites

41

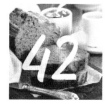

42

Coffee Cake Loaf With No-Carb Vanilla Icing

43

Chocolate Peppermint Christmas Loaf

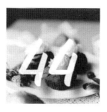

44

Holiday Spiced Chocolate Cupcakes With Buttercream Frosting

WINTER
Recipes

COLD TREATS

Walnut Parfait With Cinnamon Streusel

46

MEGA-CHOCOLATE CHUNK CHOCOLATE *Chip Cookies*

INGREDIENTS:

- 2 cups finely ground almond flour
- 2 eggs
- ½ cup butter, melted (use coconut oil for a paleo version)
- ½ cup unsweetened dark chocolate chunks
- 3 Tbsp. monk fruit sweetener
- 1 tsp. gluten- and aluminum-free baking powder
- 1 tsp. pure vanilla extract
- ½ tsp. sea salt

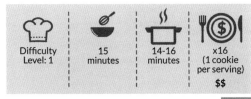

Difficulty Level: 1 | 15 minutes | 14-16 minutes | x16 (1 cookie per serving) $$

GF

DIRECTIONS:

1. Preheat the oven to 350 degrees F, and line a baking sheet with parchment paper.
2. Add the eggs, melted butter, and vanilla to a large bowl and whisk.
3. Add the rest of the ingredients and mix well.
4. Drop by the rounded tablespoon onto the parchment lined baking sheet and bake for 14-16 minutes or until the edges begin to brown.

Preparation Instructions:

You can also use 1 teaspoon of stevia in place of the monk fruit if preferred.

Serving Suggestions:

Serve with a cup of unsweetened almond milk.

Nutritional Information:

Carbs: 3g

Fiber: 1g

Net Carbs: 2g

Fat: 12g

Protein: 3g

Calories: 130

CHEWY BROWNIE MINI *Cookies*

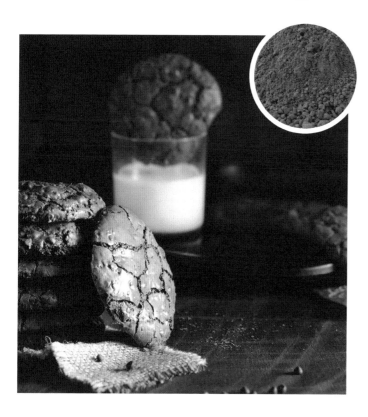

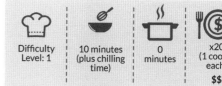

Difficulty Level: 1	10 minutes (plus chilling time)	0 minutes	x20 (1 cookie each) $$

GF

INGREDIENTS:

- ⅓ cup coconut flour, sifted
- ¼ cup raw unsweetened cocoa powder
- ½ cup raw cacao nibs
- 1 cup butter, melted (use ghee for a paleo version)
- 2 eggs
- ½ cup Swerve
- 1 tsp. pure vanilla extract
- ½ tsp. sea salt

Preparation Instructions:

You can use 1 teaspoon of stevia powder in place of the Swerve if preferred.

Serving Suggestions:

Serve with a glass of unsweetened almond or coconut milk.

DIRECTIONS:

1. Preheat the oven to 350 degrees F and line a baking sheet with parchment paper.
2. Add the melted butter, eggs, and vanilla to a large mixing bowl and whisk.
3. Add the dry ingredients and mix until no lumps remain.
4. Scoop the dough by the rounded teaspoon and bake for 10-14 minutes or until the edges begin to get crispy and the center of the cookie begins to set.

Nutritional Information:	
Carbs: 4g	**Fat:** 15g
Fiber: 3g	**Protein:** 1g
Net Carbs: 1g	**Calories:** 153

KETO GINGERBREAD
Cookies

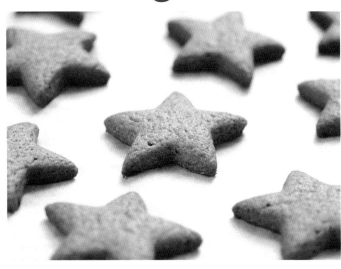

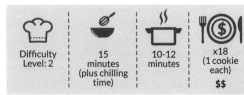

Difficulty Level: 2	15 minutes (plus chilling time)	10-12 minutes	x18 (1 cookie each) $$

GF

INGREDIENTS:

- 2 cups finely ground almond flour
- 2 eggs
- 1 cup butter, melted (use coconut or ghee for a paleo version)
- ⅓ cup monk fruit sweetener
- 1 tsp. baking powder
- 1 tsp. ground cinnamon
- ½ tsp. ground ginger
- ¼ tsp. ground nutmeg
- ⅛ tsp. ground cloves
- 1 tsp. pure vanilla extract
- ⅛ tsp. sea salt
- 1½ tsp. blackstrap molasses

Preparation Instructions:

To cream the butter, if you don't have a handheld mixer, you can add the butter to a food processor or high-speed blender.

Serving Suggestions:

Serve with a glass of unsweetened almond or coconut milk.

DIRECTIONS:

1. Preheat the oven to 350 degrees F and line a baking sheet with parchment paper.
2. Add the almond flour, spices, baking powder, and sea salt to a large mixing bowl and whisk well.
3. Cream the butter by adding it to a large mixing bowl and whipping with a handheld mixer. Add the monk fruit sweetener, molasses, and vanilla and whip again.
4. Add the eggs one at a time mixing again until combined.
5. Pour the almond flour mixture in slowly and mix with the handheld mixer until combined well.
6. Drop by rounded tablespoons onto the lined baking sheet and press down gently to flatten. For an added holiday touch use your favorite holiday-inspired cookie cutter!
7. Bake 10-12 minutes or until the edges begin to brown.
8. Allow to cool before enjoying.

Nutritional Information:	
Carbs: 5g	**Fat:** 12g
Fiber: 0g	**Protein:** 1g
Net Carbs: 5g	**Calories:** 118

SNOWFLAKE CHRISTMAS SPICE
Sugar Cookies

Difficulty Level: 2	15 minutes (plus chilling time)	7-10 minutes	x16 (1 cookie each) $$

GF

INGREDIENTS:

- 1 cup almond flour
- 2 Tbsp. coconut flour (sifted)
- ½ tsp. baking powder
- ¼ tsp. ground nutmeg
- ⅛ tsp. ground cloves
- ½ cup butter (use coconut oil or ghee for a paleo version)
- ¼ cup erythritol
- 1 tsp. pure vanilla extract
- ⅛ tsp. salt

Preparation Instructions:

To cream the butter, you can also use a handheld mixer.

Serving Suggestions:

Serve with a glass of unsweetened almond or coconut milk.

Nutritional Information:	
Carbs: 5g	Fat: 7g
Fiber: 1g	Protein: 1g
Net Carbs: 4g	Calories: 69

DIRECTIONS:

1. Preheat the oven to 350 degrees F and line a baking sheet with parchment paper.
2. Cream the butter by adding it to a food processor. Blend with the vanilla until fluffy.
3. Add the remaining dry ingredients to a large mixing bowl and stir to combine.
4. Pour dry mixture into the blender or food processor slowly and blend until combined.
5. Place the dough in the fridge for about 15 minutes.
6. Once chilled, place the dough onto the parchment-lined baking sheet and roll to about 1-inch thick on a greased surface. Alternatively, you could line another large baking sheet with parchment paper and roll the dough out on the sheet.
7. Using a snowflake cookie cutter, cut into snowflake shapes and place on the parchment-lined baking sheet.
8. Bake for 7-10 minutes or until the edges begin to brown.
9. Cool completely before enjoying!

THE ULTIMATE LOW-CARB APPLE PIE *Savory Bites*

INGREDIENTS:

- 1 cup raw cashews
- ½ cup unsweetened coconut butter
- 1 red apple, skin removed, finely chopped
- ½ tsp. ground cinnamon
- ¼ tsp. ground nutmeg
- 1 tsp. pure vanilla extract
- ¼ tsp. sea salt

Preparation Instructions:

You can also use a Granny Smith apple if preferred.

Serving Suggestions:

Serve with a cup of hot tea of coffee.

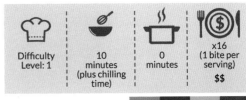

Difficulty Level: 1 | 10 minutes (plus chilling time) | 0 minutes | x16 (1 bite per serving) $$

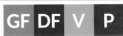

GF DF V P

DIRECTIONS:

1. Add the cashews and coconut butter to a food processor, and process until the mixture comes together.
2. Add in the remaining ingredients and blend until mixed well.
3. Place the mixture in the fridge for 10 minutes.
4. While the mixture is chilling, line a baking sheet with parchment paper.
5. Roll the chilled dough into 16 rounds and place on the lined baking sheet.
6. Refrigerate for at least 1 hour before serving.
7. Store leftovers covered in the fridge.

Nutritional Information:	
Carbs: 8g	**Fat:** 13g
Fiber: 3g	**Protein:** 2g
Net Carbs: 5g	**Calories:** 150

VALENTINE'S DAY CHOCOLATE RASPBERRY
Fat Bombs

INGREDIENTS:

- 1 cup whipped cream cheese
- 2 Tbsp. ghee
- ¼ cup unsweetened dark chocolate chips
- ¼ cup frozen raspberries
- 1 tsp. pure vanilla extract
- 10 drops liquid vanilla stevia

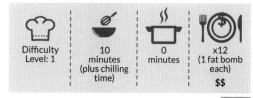

Difficulty Level: 1 | 10 minutes (plus chilling time) | 0 minutes | x12 (1 fat bomb each) $$

Preparation Instructions:

You can use butter instead of ghee if preferred.

Serving Suggestions:

Serve with a mug of hot coffee for a tasty Valentine's Day dessert.

Nutritional Information:	
Carbs: 2g	**Fat:** 12g
Fiber: 1g	**Protein:** 2g
Net Carbs: 1g	**Calories:** 122

DIRECTIONS:

1. Add the whipped cream cheese, ghee, and raspberries to a food processor or blender and blend until the mixture is mixed and "fluffy."
2. Add the vanilla extract and stevia and whip again.
3. Fold in the dark chocolate chips and then pour the mixture into silicone baking molds, filling all the way.
4. Freeze for about 1 hour before serving and store leftovers in the freezer.

DARK CHOCOLATE PEPPERMINT *Bark*

INGREDIENTS:

- ½ cup coconut oil
- ¼ cup full-fat unsweetened coconut milk
- ¼ cup raw unsweetened cocoa powder
- ½ tsp. pure peppermint extract
- ² tsp. pure vanilla extract
- ¹⁰ drops liquid vanilla stevia
- ¼ tsp. sea salt

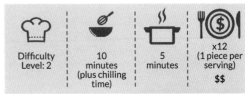

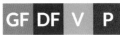

Preparation Instructions:

You can also add ¼ cup raw cocoa nibs to the chocolate mixture for added crunch.

Serving Suggestions:

Serve with a glass of unsweetened almond milk.

Nutritional Information:

Carbs: 1g	**Fat:** 11g
Fiber: 1g	**Protein:** 1g
Net Carbs: 0g	**Calories:** 94

DIRECTIONS:

1. Line a baking pan with parchment paper.
2. Add the coconut oil to a saucepan over low to medium heat and warm until melted.
3. Whisk in the coconut milk, cocoa powder, peppermint, and vanilla extract.
4. Add the stevia, and sea salt.
5. Pour the mixture into the lined baking pan and freeze for 15-20 minutes or until set.
6. Once set, slice into 12 pieces and store leftovers covered in the fridge or freezer for future use.

BLONDIES

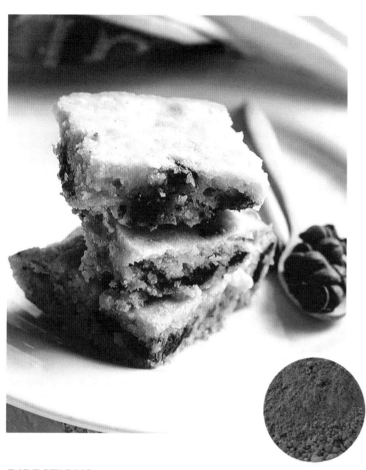

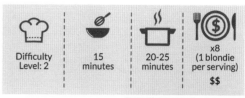

Difficulty Level: 2	15 minutes	20-25 minutes	x8 (1 blondie per serving) $$

GF **DF** **V** **P**

INGREDIENTS:

- 2 cups finely ground almond flour
- 2 eggs
- ½ cup coconut oil, melted
- 1 tsp. powdered stevia
- 1 tsp. pure vanilla extract
- ½ cup of unsweetened dark chocolate chips
- 1 tsp. gluten- and aluminum-free baking powder

Preparation Instructions:

If you cannot find unsweetened chocolate chips, you can also use raw cocoa nibs.

Serving Suggestions:

Serve with a dollop of unsweetened whipped cream if desired.

DIRECTIONS:

1. Preheat the oven to 350 degrees F, and line a 9x13-inch baking pan with parchment paper.
2. Add eggs to a mixing bowl and whisk.
3. Mix in the coconut oil, vanilla extract, and stevia. Mix well.
4. Fold in the almond flour, baking powder, and dark chocolate chips.
5. Pour the mixture into the lined baking pan and bake for 20-25 minutes or until the edges begin to brown.
6. Cool, and then slice into 8 squares.

Nutritional Information:

Carbs: 6g	**Fat:** 26g
Fiber: 3g	**Protein:** 5g
Net Carbs: 3g	**Calories:** 275

EGGNOG *Brownies*

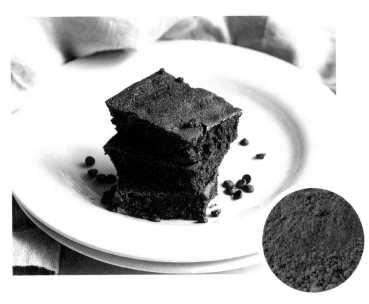

Difficulty Level: 2	15 minutes	20-25 minutes	x8 (1 brownie per serving) $$

INGREDIENTS:

- 2 cups finely ground almond flour
- 2 eggs
- ½ cup coconut oil, melted
- ¼ cup raw unsweetened cocoa powder
- ¼ cup unsweetened dark chocolate chips
- 1 tsp. powdered stevia
- 1 tsp. pure vanilla extract
- 1 tsp. ground cinnamon
- ½ tsp. ground nutmeg
- 1 tsp. gluten- and aluminum-free baking powder
- ⅛ tsp. sea salt
- 2 Tbsp. water

DIRECTIONS:

1. Preheat the oven to 350 degrees F, and line a 9x13-inch baking pan with parchment paper.
2. Add the eggs to a mixing bowl and whisk.
3. Mix in the coconut oil, vanilla extract, and stevia. Mix well.
4. Add the almond flour, baking powder, cocoa powder, cinnamon, nutmeg, sea salt, and water. Mix well.
5. Fold in the chocolate chips, pour the mixture into the lined baking pan and bake for 20-25 minutes or until a toothpick inserted into the center comes out clean.
6. Cool, and then slice into 8 squares.

Preparation Instructions:

If you are not avoiding dairy, you can use butter instead of coconut oil if preferred.

Serving Suggestions:

Serve with a dollop of unsweetened whipped cream if desired.

Nutritional Information:

Carbs: 6g

Fiber: 3g

Net Carbs: 3g

Fat: 23g

Protein: 4g

Calories: 233

CHRISTMAS-INSPIRED PECAN PIE *Savory Bites*

INGREDIENTS:

- 1 cup raw pecans
- ½ cup shredded unsweetened coconut
- 2 Tbsp. coconut butter
- 1 tsp. pure vanilla extract
- 10 drops liquid vanilla stevia
- 1 tsp. ground cinnamon
- ¼ tsp. allspice
- ¼ cup raw cacao nibs

Difficulty Level: 2	10 minutes (plus chilling time)	0 minutes	x12 (1 bite per serving) $$

DIRECTIONS:

1. Add the pecans and shredded coconut to a high-speed blender or food processor and blend until combined well.
2. Add the coconut butter, vanilla, stevia, cinnamon, and allspice and blend again.
3. Pour the mixture into a mixing bowl and fold in the cacao nibs.
4. Refrigerate to chill for 15 minutes.
5. Once chilled, roll into bite-sized rounds.
6. Store leftovers covered in the fridge.

Preparation Instructions:

You can use raw walnuts or cashews in place of the pecans if preferred.

Serving Suggestions:

Serve with a mug of keto eggnog for a holiday treat.

Nutritional Information:

Carbs: 8g

Fiber: 6g

Net Carbs: 2g

Fat: 30g

Protein: 3g

Calories: 298

COFFEE CAKE LOAF WITH NO-CARB *Vanilla Icing*

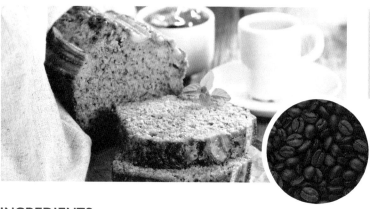

Difficulty Level: 2 | 20 minutes | 20-30 minutes | x8 (1 slice per serving) $$

GF

INGREDIENTS:

- 2½ cups almond flour
- ½ cup brewed coffee, chilled
- 3 eggs
- ½ cup ghee, melted
- 1 tsp. powdered stevia
- 1 tsp. ground cinnamon
- 1 tsp. pure vanilla extract

No-Carb Vanilla Icing:

- 1 cup whipped cream cheese
- ¼ cup heavy whipping cream
- 1 tsp. liquid vanilla cream stevia
- 1 tsp. pure vanilla extract

Preparation Instructions:

To make this paleo-friendly, try using almond-based cream cheese and full-fat unsweetened coconut cream.

Serving Suggestions:

Serve with a mug of keto hot chocolate or a hot cup of coffee.

DIRECTIONS:

1. Line a loaf pan with parchment paper and preheat the oven to 325 degrees F.
2. Add the eggs to a mixing bowl and whisk.
3. Add the ghee, vanilla extract, and coffee and whisk again.
4. Add the dry ingredients and whisk until no lumps remain.
5. Bake for 20-30 minutes or until a toothpick inserted into the center comes out clean.
6. While the loaf is baking, make the frosting by adding the ingredients to a food processor, and whip until creamy.
7. Once the loaf is cool, top with the frosting, slice into 8 even pieces and enjoy!

Nutritional Information:

Carbs: 6g	**Fat:** 19g
Fiber: 1g	**Protein:** 6g
Net Carbs: 5g	**Calories:** 218

CHOCOLATE PEPPERMINT
Christmas Loaf

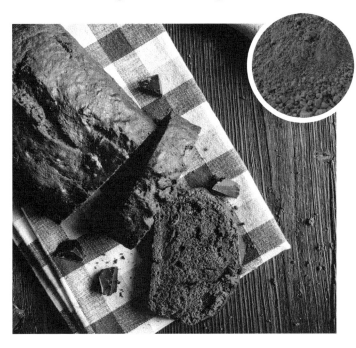

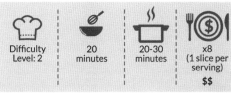

Difficulty Level: 2	20 minutes	20-30 minutes	x8 (1 slice per serving) $$

GF

INGREDIENTS:

- 2½ cups almond flour
- ¼ cup raw unsweetened cocoa powder
- ½ cup unsweetened almond milk
- 3 eggs
- ½ cup butter, melted (use ghee for a paleo version)
- 1 tsp. powdered stevia
- 1 tsp. pure peppermint extract
- ¼ cup unsweetened dark chocolate chips

Preparation Instructions:

Feel free to add some additional holiday flair by including 1 teaspoon ground nutmeg if desired.

Serving Suggestions:

Serve with a mug of tea or hot coffee.

DIRECTIONS:

1. Line a loaf pan with parchment paper and preheat the oven to 325 degrees F.
2. Add the eggs to mixing bowl and whisk.
3. Add the butter, peppermint, and almond milk, and whisk again.
4. Add all the dry ingredients and whisk until no lumps remain.
5. Bake for 20-30 minutes or until a toothpick inserted into the center comes out clean.
6. Allow the loaf to cool for 10 minutes. Slice and enjoy!

Nutritional Information:	
Carbs: 6g	**Fat:** 22g
Fiber: 3g	**Protein:** 6g
Net Carbs: 3g	**Calories:** 234

HOLIDAY SPICED CHOCOLATE CUPCAKES WITH *Buttercream Frosting*

INGREDIENTS:

- 1 cup coconut flour
- ½ cup unsweetened cocoa powder
- 1 tsp. powdered stevia
- 3 eggs
- 1 cup half and half
- ½ cup butter, melted
- 2 tsp. pure vanilla extract
- 2 tsp. baking powder
- 1 tsp. ground cinnamon
- ½ tsp. ground nutmeg

Buttercream Frosting

- ½ cup butter
- ½ cup whipped cream cheese
- 2 tsp. Pure vanilla extract
- 2 drops of liquid vanilla stevia (optional)

Difficulty Level: 1	15 minutes	18-20 minutes	x16 (1 cupcake per serving) $$

Cooking tip:

Coconut flour is very absorbent, so the batter will be thicker than traditional cake batter. Instead of pouring the mixture into the muffin tin, scoop with a spoon and gently press down to flatten.

DIRECTIONS:

1. Start by preheating the oven to 350 degrees F and lining a muffin tin with liners.
2. Add all of the dry ingredients to one bowl and mix well.
3. In a separate bowl, whisk the eggs. Mix in the half and half, melted butter, and pure vanilla extract.
4. Pour the wet mixture into the dry and stir until well-combined and until no clumps remain.
5. Scoop the cupcake batter into the lined muffin tins, filling ¾ of the way.
6. Bake at 350 for 18-20 minutes.
7. Cool completely before frosting with the buttercream frosting.

Buttercream Frosting Directions:

1. Add all the frosting ingredients to a large bowl and cream using a hand-held mixture. Alternatively, use a food processor and whip until well combined.
2. Transfer the mixture to a piping bag, and frost each cupcake once completely cool.

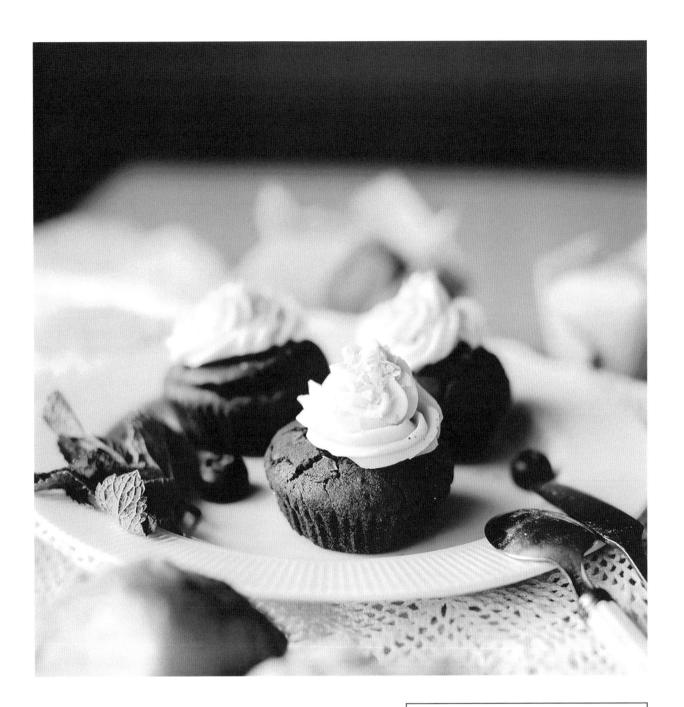

Nutritional Information:

Carbs: 12g   **Fat:** 18g

Fiber: 7g   **Protein:** 4g

Net Carbs: 5g   **Calories:** 226

WALNUT PARFAIT WITH CINNAMON

Streusel

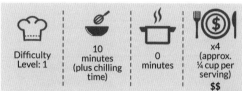

GF

INGREDIENTS:

- 1 cup full-fat unsweetened Greek yogurt (use full-fat unsweetened coconut milk yogurt for a paleo version)
- ¼ cup chopped walnuts
- 1 tsp. pure vanilla extract
- ½ tsp. ground cinnamon

Cinnamon Streusel:

- 3 Tbsp. coconut oil
- ½ cup chopped walnuts
- 1 tsp. Swerve sweetener
- 2 tsp. ground cinnamon

DIRECTIONS:

1. Add yogurt to the base of a serving bowl and stir in the vanilla and cinnamon.
2. Top with the chopped walnuts and set aside.
3. Make the cinnamon streusel by adding all the ingredients to a mixing bowl and mix well.
4. Add the cinnamon streusel on top of the yogurt bowl and enjoy!

Preparation Instructions:

You can make this parfait using pecans if preferred.

Serving Suggestions:

Enjoy with a dollop of unsweetened whipped cream if desired.

Nutritional Information:

Carbs: 8g

Fiber: 3g

Net Carbs: 5g

Fat: 30g

Protein: 9g

Calories: 313

SPRING
Recipes

SAVORY BITES & CHOCOLATES

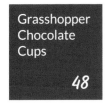
Grasshopper Chocolate Cups
48

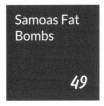
Samoas Fat Bombs
49

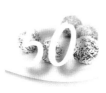
50

Easter Day Carrot Cake Fat Bombs

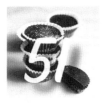
51

Almond Butter Cups

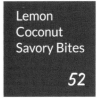
Lemon Coconut Savory Bites
52

BROWNIES & CAKE

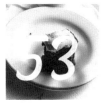
53

Saint Patrick's Day Brownies

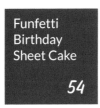
Funfetti Birthday Sheet Cake
54

COLD TREATS

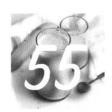
55

Sea Salt Vanilla Almond Butter Milkshake

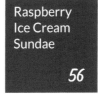
Raspberry Ice Cream Sundae
56

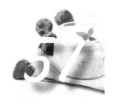
57

Strawberry Mint Frozen Yogurt

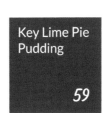
58

Easter-Inspired Coconut Cream Pie Pudding

Key Lime Pie Pudding
59

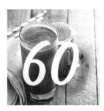
60

Pistachio Brownie Batter Milkshake

GRASSHOPPER CHOCOLATE *Cups*

INGREDIENTS:

- 1 cup unsweetened dark chocolate chips
- 2 Tbsp. coconut oil
- 1 tsp. pure peppermint extract
- 10 drops liquid stevia
- ½ tsp. sea salt

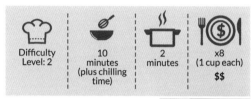

Difficulty Level: 2 | 10 minutes (plus chilling time) | 2 minutes | x8 (1 cup each) $$

GF DF P

DIRECTIONS:

1. Add mini muffin tin liners to a baking sheet and set aside.
2. Make the chocolate coating by adding the coconut oil to a stockpot over low heat. Melt the oil and then add the chocolate chips and salt.
3. Stir the mixture continuously until completely melted.
4. Stir in the peppermint extract and stevia.
5. Pour the mixture into the mini muffin liners, filling about ¾ of the way.
6. Freeze for about 15 minutes or until set.
7. Store leftovers in the fridge or freezer.

Preparation Instructions:

You can replace the peppermint extract and use vanilla or almond extract instead if desired.

Serving Suggestions:

Serve with a cup of unsweetened almond milk.

> **Nutritional Information:**
> **Carbs:** 8g
> **Fiber:** 4g
> **Net Carbs:** 4g
> **Fat:** 19g
> **Protein:** 4g
> **Calories:** 231

SAMOAS FAT *Bombs*

INGREDIENTS:

- 1 cup raw cashews
- 2 Tbsp. butter (use ghee for a paleo version)
- 2 Tbsp. unsweetened coconut butter
- 1 Tbsp. Swerve sweetener (use coconut sugar for a paleo option)
- 2 Tbsp. unsweetened coconut cream
- 1 tsp. pure vanilla extract
- 1 tsp. blackstrap molasses
- ½ tsp. sea salt
- ½ cup shredded unsweetened coconut

Difficulty Level: 1	15 minutes (plus chilling time)	0 minutes	x20 (1 fat bomb each) $$

DIRECTIONS:

1. Line a baking sheet with parchment paper and add the shredded unsweetened coconut to a large bowl. Set aside.
2. Add the cashews, butter, and coconut butter to a high-speed blender or food processor, and process until the cashews are ground finely.
3. Add the Swerve, coconut cream, vanilla, molasses, and salt and blend again.
4. Form into 20 bite-sized rounds and roll into the shredded unsweetened coconut.
5. Place on the parchment lined baking sheet and set in the fridge for 30 minutes before enjoying.
6. Store leftovers covered in the fridge or the freezer.

Preparation Instructions:

If you are in a pinch, you can freeze the fat bombs for 15 minutes or refrigerate for 30 minutes.

Serving Suggestions:

Serve with a cup of coffee or tea.

Nutritional Information:

Carbs: 6g

Fiber: 1g

Net Carbs: 5g

Fat: 11g

Protein: 2g

Calories: 120

EASTER DAY CARROT CAKE FAT *Bombs*

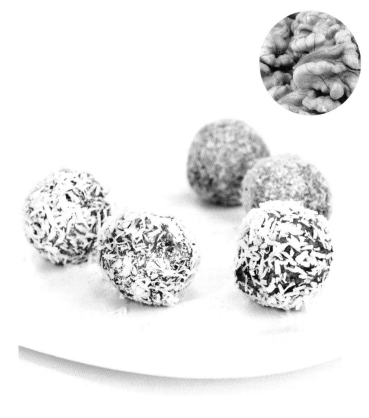

| Difficulty Level: 1 | 15 minutes (plus chilling time) | 0 minutes | x14 (1 fat bomb per serving) $$ |

GF **V** **P**

INGREDIENTS:

- 1 cup walnuts
- 1 cup unsweetened coconut butter
- ½ cup shredded carrots
- ½ cup shredded unsweetened coconut
- 1 tsp. powdered stevia
- 1 tsp. pure vanilla extract
- 1 tsp. ground cinnamon
- ⅛ tsp. ground nutmeg
- ⅛ tsp. ground ginger

Preparation Instructions:

You can use pecans or cashews in place of the walnuts if preferred.

Serving Suggestions:

Serve with a cup of tea for a tasty Easter dessert treat.

DIRECTIONS:

1. Add walnuts, coconut butter, shredded carrots, and half of the shredded coconut to a food processor or high-speed blender and blend until combined well.
2. Add in the remaining ingredients minus the shredded coconut, and blend until combined.
3. Chill for 15 minutes in the fridge.
4. Roll into bite-sized rounds and roll into the remaining shredded unsweetened coconut.
5. Enjoy and store leftovers in the fridge or the freezer.

Nutritional Information:	
Carbs: 11g	**Fat:** 29g
Fiber: 6g	**Protein:** 5g
Net Carbs: 5g	**Calories:** 320

ALMOND BUTTER *Cups*

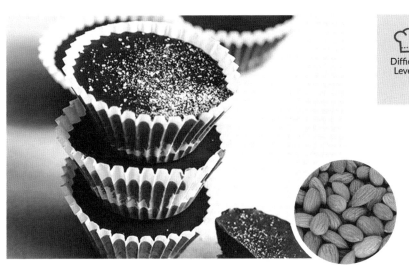

Difficulty Level: 2	20 minutes (plus chilling time)	3 minutes	x10 (1 almond butter cup each) $$

GF DF P

INGREDIENTS:

Chocolate Coating:
- 1 cup unsweetened dark chocolate chips
- 2 Tbsp. coconut oil
- ½ tsp. sea salt

Almond Butter Filling:
- ¼ cup unsweetened almond butter
- 1 tsp. powdered stevia
- 1 tsp. pure vanilla extract
- 1 Tbsp. coconut flour

Nutritional Information:

Carbs: 9g **Fat:** 19g

Fiber: 4g **Protein:** 4g

Net Carbs: 5g **Calories:** 230

DIRECTIONS:

1. Add mini muffin tin liners to a baking sheet and set aside.
2. Make the chocolate coating by adding the coconut oil to a stockpot over low heat. Melt the oil and then add the chocolate chips and salt.
3. Stir the mixture continuously until completely melted.
4. Once melted, scoop about 1 teaspoon of the chocolate mixture into the mini muffin liners to cover the bottom. Place in the freezer for about 15 minutes or until set.
5. While the chocolate is setting, make the almond butter filling by adding the almond butter, vanilla, and stevia to a mixing bowl and stir.
6. Add the coconut flour and mix well.
7. Once hardened, add about a teaspoon of the almond butter filling to the mini muffin liners and top with about 2 more teaspoons of the melted chocolate mixture.
8. Freeze for another 15-20 minutes or until hardened.
9. Store in the fridge or freezer until ready to enjoy.

LEMON COCONUT
Savory Bites

INGREDIENTS:

- 1 cup cream cheese
- 4 Tbsp. ghee, softened
- 10 drops liquid stevia
- 1 Tbsp. freshly squeezed lemon juice
- ½ cup shredded unsweetened coconut

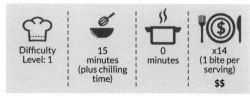

DIRECTIONS:

1. Add cream cheese, ghee, and stevia to a high-speed blender or food processor and whip until the mixture is fluffy.
2. Add the lemon juice and whip again.
3. Scoop the mixture into silicone mini cupcake molds and sprinkle with the shredded coconut.
4. Freeze for about 1 hour before enjoying.
5. Store leftovers in the freezer.

Preparation Instructions:

You can use butter instead of ghee if preferred.

Serving Suggestions:

Serve with a dollop of whipped cream if desired.

Nutritional Information:

Carbs: 1g

Fiber: 0g

Net Carbs: 1g

Fat: 10g

Protein: 1g

Calories: 100

SAINT PATRICK'S DAY *Brownies*

Difficulty Level: 2	15 minutes	30-35 minutes	x8 (1 brownie per serving) $$

GF

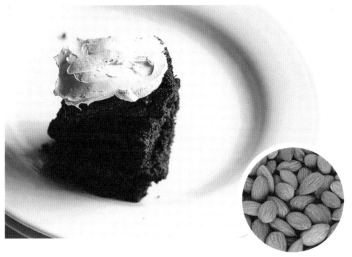

INGREDIENTS:

- 2 cups almond flour
- 2 eggs
- 1 stick butter, melted (use coconut oil for a paleo version)
- ¼ cup raw unsweetened cocoa powder
- 1 tsp. pure peppermint extract
- 1 tsp. stevia powder
- 1 tsp. gluten- and aluminum-free baking powder
- ⅛ tsp. sea salt
- 2 Tbsp. water

Mint Frosting:

- 1 cup whipped cream cheese (use full-fat unsweetened coconut cream for a paleo version)
- 1 drop liquid stevia
- 1 tsp. plant-based green food coloring (artificial coloring-free)

DIRECTIONS:

1. Preheat the oven to 350 degrees F and line a 9x13-inch baking pan with parchment paper.
2. Add the eggs to a mixing bowl and whisk.
3. Mix in the butter, peppermint extract, and stevia. Mix well.
4. Add the almond flour, baking powder, sea salt, and water. Mix well.
5. Pour the mixture into the lined baking pan and bake for 30-35 minutes or until a toothpick inserted into the center comes out clean.
6. While the brownies are baking, make the peppermint frosting by adding the whipped cream cheese to a mixing bowl with the green food coloring, peppermint extract, and stevia. Using a handheld mixer, whip until a fluffy consistency forms.
7. Once the brownies are cooled, top with the frosting, and then slice into 8 squares.
8. Store leftovers in the fridge.

Preparation Instructions:

You can add ¼ cup of unsweetened dark chocolate chips to the batter for an added savory taste.

Serving Suggestions:

Serve with a mug of coffee or tea.

Nutritional Information:	
Carbs: 5g	**Fat:** 17g
Fiber: 2g	**Protein:** 8g
Net Carbs: 3g	**Calories:** 192

FUNFETTI BIRTHDAY SHEET *Cake*

INGREDIENTS:

For Sprinkles:

- ½ cup shredded unsweetened coconut
- Assortment of plant-based food coloring colors

For Cake:

- 2 cups finely ground almond flour
- 2 eggs
- 2 cups whipped cream cheese
- ¼ cup unsweetened almond milk
- 1 stick butter, melted
- 1 tsp. pure vanilla extract
- ¼ cup Swerve
- 1 tsp. baking powder
- Coconut oil for greasing

For Whipped Cream:

- 2 cups heavy whipping cream
- 1 drop liquid stevia
- 1 tsp. pure vanilla extract

Preparation Instructions:

Feel free to use whatever low-calorie sweetener you prefer in the cake recipe.

Serving Suggestions:

Serve with a glass of unsweetened almond milk.

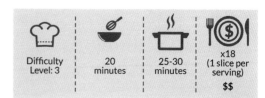

Difficulty Level: 3 | 20 minutes | 25-30 minutes | x18 (1 slice per serving) $$

DIRECTIONS:

1. Preheat the oven to 350 degrees F and grease a large cake pan with coconut oil.
2. Make the funfetti sprinkles by dividing the shredded coconut into as many different bowls as you would like, depending on how many colors you choose to use. Use about 3-4 drops of food coloring per bowl and stir to coat the shredded coconut completely. Set aside.
3. Add the almond flour, Swerve, and baking powder to a bowl. Whisk to combine and then set aside.
4. In a separate bowl, add the eggs, melted butter, whipped cream cheese, vanilla, and almond milk and whisk well.
5. Pour the dry mixture into the egg mixture and stir until combined well.
6. Fold in the sprinkles and stir well.
7. Pour the mixture into the cake pan and bake for 25-30 minutes or until a toothpick inserted into the center comes out clean.
8. While the cake is baking, make the whipped cream by adding all the ingredients to a food processor and blend until a whipped cream-like consistency forms. Store in the fridge until ready to use.
9. Allow the cake to cool, and then serve with whipped cream immediately before serving.

Nutritional Information:

Carbs: 6g   **Fat:** 22g

Fiber: 1g   **Protein:** 4g

Net Carbs: 5g   **Calories:** 216

SEA SALT VANILLA ALMOND BUTTER
Milkshake

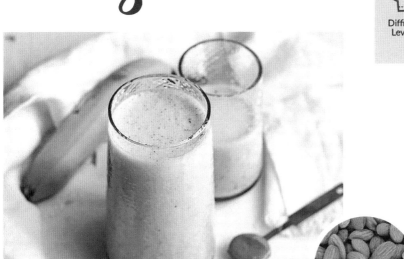

Difficulty Level: 1	5 minutes	0 minutes	x2 (about ½ cup per serving) $$

GF DF P

DIRECTIONS:

1. Add all ingredients to a high-speed blender and blend until smooth.
2. Enjoy right away.

Preparation Instructions:

If you are not avoiding dairy, you can use ½ cup of heavy cream and 1 cup of whole milk in this recipe.

Serving Suggestions:

Serve with a dollop of unsweetened whipped cream if desired.

INGREDIENTS:

- 1 cup unsweetened almond milk
- 2 Tbsp. almond butter
- 1 tsp. pure vanilla extract
- 1 drop liquid vanilla cream stevia
- 1 pinch of sea salt

Nutritional Information:	
Carbs: 4g	**Fat:** 11g
Fiber: 2g	**Protein:** 4g
Net Carbs: 2g	**Calories:** 124

RASPBERRY ICE CREAM *Sundae*

INGREDIENTS:

- 1 can unsweetened full-fat coconut cream
- ¼ cup frozen raspberries
- 1 tsp. pure vanilla extract
- 1 tsp. liquid stevia

Toppings:
- 4 Tbsp. sugar-free chocolate syrup
- ¼ cup walnut pieces

DIRECTIONS:

1. Add the coconut cream, raspberries, vanilla, and stevia to a high-speed blender, and blend until smooth.
2. Top with the sugar-free chocolate syrup and walnut pieces and serve.

Preparation Instructions:

You can use strawberries in place of raspberries if preferred.

Serving Suggestions:

Serve with a dollop of whipped cream if desired.

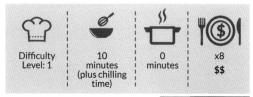

Difficulty Level: 1 | 10 minutes (plus chilling time) | 0 minutes | x8 $$

GF DF P

Nutritional Information:

Carbs: 6g

Fiber: 1g

Net Carbs: 5g

Fat: 15g

Protein: 3g

Calories: 170

STRAWBERRY MINT *Yogurt*

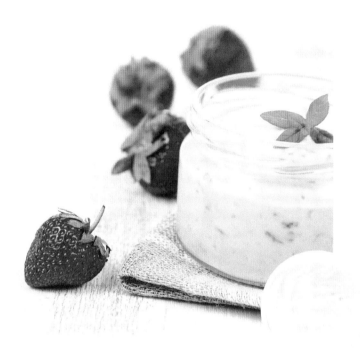

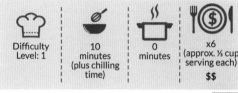

Difficulty Level: 1	10 minutes (plus chilling time)	0 minutes	x6 (approx. ⅓ cup serving each) $$

GF

INGREDIENTS:

- 2 cups full-fat unsweetened Greek yogurt (use full-fat unsweetened coconut milk yogurt for a paleo version)
- 1 cup strawberries
- 1 tsp. freshly chopped mint leaves
- 1 tsp. pure vanilla extract

DIRECTIONS:

1. Add all the ingredients to a high-speed blender, and blend until smooth.
2. Chill in the fridge for 1 hour before serving.
3. Enjoy, and store leftovers covered in the fridge.

Preparation Instructions:

You can use raspberries or blueberries in this recipe if preferred.

Serving Suggestions:

Serve with a dollop of whipped cream if desired.

Nutritional Information:

Carbs: 5g

Fiber: 1g

Net Carbs: 4g

Fat: 3g

Protein: 7g

Calories: 80

EASTER-INSPIRED COCONUT CREAM
Pie Pudding

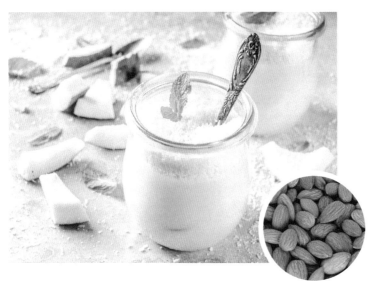

Difficulty Level: 1	15 minutes (plus chilling time)	0 minutes	x6 (approx. ½ cup per serving) $$

GF

INGREDIENTS:

- 2 cups full-fat unsweetened coconut milk
- 1 cup heavy cream (use another 1 cup of full-fat unsweetened coconut milk for a paleo version)
- 2 Tbsp. ghee, melted
- ½ cup erythritol
- 1 cup shredded unsweetened coconut, divided
- 1 tsp. pure vanilla extract

DIRECTIONS:

1. Add the coconut milk, heavy cream, vanilla, and melted ghee to a food processor, and blend until smooth.
2. Add the erythritol and ½ cup of shredded coconut.
3. Chill for 1 hour.
4. Once chilled, divide among 6 cups and top with additional shredded coconut and serve.

Preparation Instructions:

Feel free to use 1 drop of liquid stevia in place of the erythritol if preferred.

Serving Suggestions:

Serve with a dollop of whipped cream if desired.

Nutritional Information:

Carbs: 7g

Fiber: 3g

Net Carbs: 4g

Fat: 35g

Protein: 3g

Calories: 340

KEY LIME PIE *Pudding*

INGREDIENTS:

- 1 cup full-fat unsweetened coconut milk
- 2 Tbsp. sour cream (use coconut cream for a paleo version)
- 1 Tbsp. erythritol (use pure maple syrup for a paleo version)
- ¼ cup freshly squeezed lime juice
- 1 tsp. pure vanilla extract
- ½ cup shredded unsweetened coconut
- 1 cup of walnuts, processed into crumbs

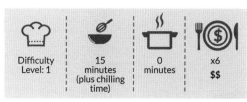

| Difficulty Level: 1 | 15 minutes (plus chilling time) | 0 minutes | x6 $$ |

GF

DIRECTIONS:

1. Start by adding the walnuts to a food processor and blend just until crumbled. Set aside.
2. Add all ingredients minus the shredded unsweetened coconut to a blender or food processor and blend until creamy.
3. Split the crumbled walnuts to the bottom of 6 serving bowls and then evenly divide the key lime mixture among the bowls.
4. Top with shredded coconut.
5. Chill for 30 minutes before serving.

Preparation Instructions:

You can use cream cheese in place of sour cream if preferred.

Serving Suggestions:

Serve with a dollop of whipped cream if desired.

Nutritional Information:

Carbs: 8g

Fiber: 3g

Net Carbs: 5g

Fat: 25g

Protein: 6g

Calories: 255

PISTACHIO BROWNIE BATTER *Milkshake*

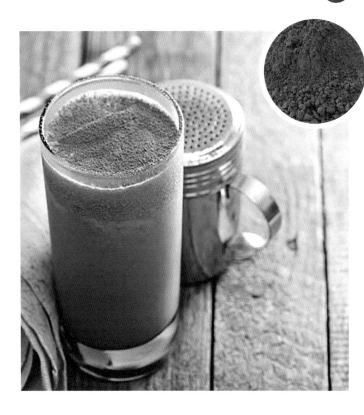

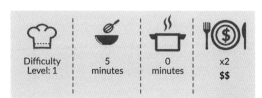

Difficulty Level: 1 | 5 minutes | 0 minutes | x2 $$

GF

INGREDIENTS:

- ½ cup heavy cream (use coconut milk for a paleo version)
- ½ cup unsweetened almond milk
- 3 drops liquid stevia
- 2 Tbsp. raw unsweetened cocoa powder
- 1 Tbsp. raw cocoa nibs
- 2 Tbsp. roasted unsalted pistachios

DIRECTIONS:

1. Add all ingredients to a high-speed blender and blend until smooth.
2. Serve right away.

Preparation Instructions:

You can use any low-carb sweetener of choice.

Serving Suggestions:

Serve with a dollop of whipped cream if desired.

Nutritional Information:

Carbs: 6g

Fiber: 3g

Net Carbs: 3g

Fat: 16g

Protein: 3g

Calories: 165

SUMMER
Recipes

FAT BOMBS & MOUSSE

Frozen Cookie Dough Fat Bombs
62

Frozen Super Chunk Brownie Fat Bombs

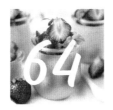

Strawberry Mousse

COLD TREATS

Super Creamy Chocolate Peanut Butter Milkshake
65

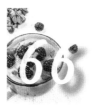

Decadent Blackberry Ice Cream

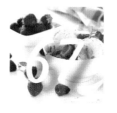

Raspberries & Cream Ice Cream

Vegan Blueberry Frozen "Yogurt"
68

Strawberries & Cream Frozen "Yogurt" Popsicles
69

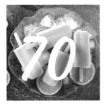

Orange Creamsicles

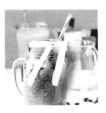

Savory Mocha Milkshake

Coconut Chocolate Chip Popsicles

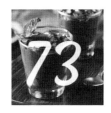

Chocolate & Almond Mint Pudding

Homemade Strawberry Whipped Cream Parfait
74

FROZEN COOKIE DOUGH *Fat Bombs*

INGREDIENTS:

- 1 cup raw cashews
- ½ cup coconut butter
- 1 tsp. pure vanilla extract
- 10 drops liquid vanilla stevia
- ¼ tsp. sea salt
- 4 Tbsp. unsweetened dark chocolate chips

Difficulty Level: 1 | 10 minutes (plus chilling time) | 0 minutes | x14 (1 fat bomb per serving) $$

GF DF P

DIRECTIONS:

1. Add raw cashews and coconut butter to a food processor or high-speed blender and blend until the cashews are ground finely.
2. Add the vanilla, stevia, and salt and blend until combined.
3. Fold in the dark chocolate chips.
4. Freeze for 20 minutes and then roll into bite-sized rounds.
5. Store in the fridge or freezer until ready to enjoy.

Preparation Instructions:

You can use raw cocoa nibs in place of the dark chocolate chips is preferred.

Serving Suggestions:

Top each fat bomb with a dollop of unsweetened whipped cream if desired.

Nutritional Information:

Carbs: 9g

Fiber: 4g

Net Carbs: 5g

Fat: 19g

Protein: 3g

Calories: 206

FROZEN SUPER CHUNK BROWNIE *Fat Bombs*

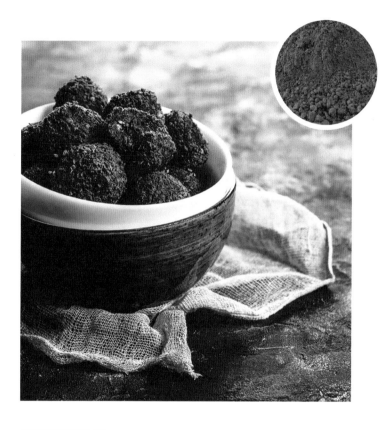

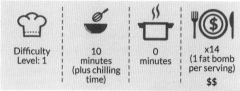

Difficulty Level: 1	10 minutes (plus chilling time)	0 minutes	x14 (1 fat bomb per serving) $$

GF DF P

INGREDIENTS:

- 1 cup raw almonds
- 2 Tbsp. raw unsweetened cocoa powder
- ½ cup coconut butter
- 1 tsp. pure vanilla extract
- 10 drops liquid vanilla stevia
- ¼ tsp. sea salt
- 4 Tbsp. unsweetened dark chocolate chips

Preparation Instructions:

You can use raw cocoa nibs in place of the dark chocolate chips is preferred.

Serving Suggestions:

Top each fat bomb with a dollop of unsweetened whipped cream if desired.

DIRECTIONS:

1. Add raw almonds and coconut butter to a food processor or high-speed blender and blend until the almonds are ground finely.
2. Add the vanilla, stevia, and salt and blend until combined.
3. Fold in the dark chocolate chips.
4. Freeze for 20 minutes and then roll into bite-sized rounds.
5. Store in the fridge or freezer until ready to enjoy.

Nutritional Information:	
Carbs: 8g	**Fat:** 18g
Fiber: 5g	**Protein:** 3g
Net Carbs: 3g	**Calories:** 191

STRAWBERRY
Mousse

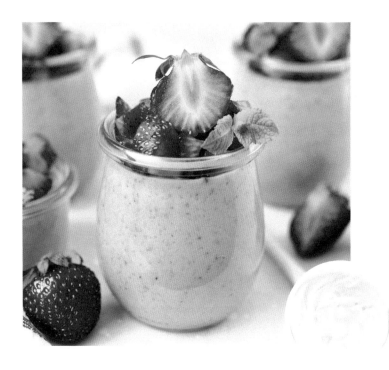

Difficulty Level: 1 | 10 minutes (plus chilling time) | 0 minutes | x4 (approx. ½ cup per serving) $$

GF

INGREDIENTS:

- 1 cup full-fat unsweetened coconut milk
- 1 cup heavy cream
- ½ cup frozen strawberries
- 1 tsp. pure vanilla extract
- 2 tsp. Swerve
- 1 Tbsp. freshly squeezed lemon juice

DIRECTIONS:

1. Add all the ingredients to a blender or food processor, and blend until creamy.
2. Divide among 4 bowls and chill for 1 hour before serving.
3. Chill for 30 minutes before serving.

Preparation Instructions:

You can use an additional 1 cup of coconut milk in place of the heavy cream if you are avoiding dairy.

Serving Suggestions:

Serve with unsweetened shredded coconut if desired.

Nutritional Information:

Carbs: 5g

Fiber: 0g

Net Carbs: 5g

Fat: 15g

Protein: 1g

Calories: 148

SUPER CREAMY CHOCOLATE PEANUT BUTTER *Milkshake*

INGREDIENTS:

- ½ cup unsweetened almond milk
- ¼ cup coconut milk
- 1 Tbsp. raw cacao powder
- 2 Tbsp. peanut butter
- 3 drops liquid stevia
- 1 tsp. pure vanilla extract

Difficulty Level: 1	5 minutes	0 minutes	x2 (about ½ cup per serving) $$

DIRECTIONS:

1. Add all ingredients to a high-speed blender, and blend until smooth.
2. Serve right away.

Preparation Instructions:

If you are not avoiding dairy, you can use ½ cup of heavy cream and 1 cup of whole milk in this recipe.

Serving Suggestions:

Serve with a dollop of unsweetened whipped cream if desired.

Nutritional Information:

Carbs: 7g

Fiber: 3g

Net Carbs: 4g

Fat: 16g

Protein: 5g

Calories: 185

DECADENT BLACKBERRY
Ice Cream (NO CHURN)

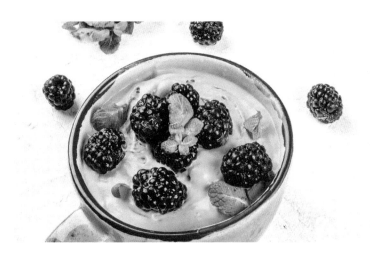

INGREDIENTS:

- 1 cup heavy cream
- 1 cup sour cream
- ½ cup frozen blackberries
- 10 drops liquid vanilla stevia

DIRECTIONS:

1. Add all ingredients to a high-speed blender, and blend until smooth.
2. Pour into a large plastic container and freeze for about 4 hours or until solid.
3. Let sit at room temperature for a few minutes before serving.

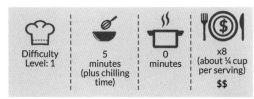

Difficulty Level: 1	5 minutes (plus chilling time)	0 minutes	x8 (about ¼ cup per serving) $$

GF

Preparation Instructions:

Feel free to use any berry of choice in this recipe.

Serving Suggestions:

Serve with a dollop of unsweetened whipped cream if desired.

Nutritional Information:

Carbs: 3g   **Fat:** 12g

Fiber: 1g   **Protein:** 1g

Net Carbs: 2g   **Calories:** 117

RASPBERRIES & CREAM
Ice Cream (NO CHURN)

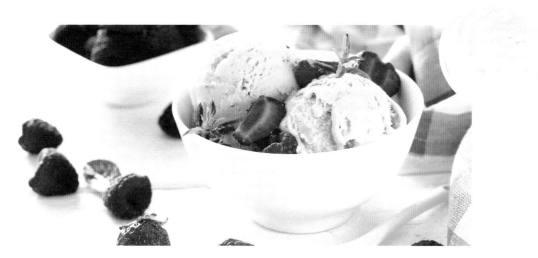

INGREDIENTS:

- 1 cup heavy cream
- 1 cup whipped cream cheese
- ½ cup frozen raspberries
- 10 drops liquid vanilla stevia
- 1 tsp. pure vanilla extract

DIRECTIONS:

1. Add all ingredients to a high-speed blender, and blend until smooth.
2. Pour into a large plastic container and freeze for about 4 hours or until solid.
3. Let sit at room temperature for a few minutes before serving.

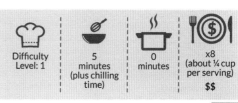

| Difficulty Level: 1 | 5 minutes (plus chilling time) | 0 minutes | x8 (about ¼ cup per serving) $$ |

GF

Preparation Instructions:

Feel free to use any berries of choice in this recipe.

Serving Suggestions:

Serve with a dollop of unsweetened whipped cream if desired.

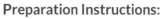

Nutritional Information:

Carbs: 5g	**Fat:** 16g
Fiber: 1g	**Protein:** 3g
Net Carbs: 4g	**Calories:** 171

VEGAN BLUEBERRY FROZEN *"Yogurt"*

INGREDIENTS:

- 2 cans unsweetened coconut cream
- ½ cup frozen blueberries
- 10 drops liquid vanilla stevia
- 1 tsp. pure vanilla extract

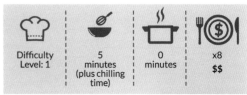

Difficulty Level: 1   5 minutes (plus chilling time)   0 minutes   x8 $$

GF DF P

DIRECTIONS:

1. Add all ingredients to a high-speed blender, and blend until smooth.
2. Pour into a large plastic container and freeze for about 4 hours or until solid.
3. Let sit at room temperature for a few minutes before serving.

Preparation Instructions:

Feel free to use any berries of choice in this recipe.

Serving Suggestions:

Serve with a dollop of unsweetened whipped cream if desired.

Nutritional Information:

Carbs: 4g

Fiber: 1g

Net Carbs: 3g

Fat: 26g

Protein: 3g

Calories: 255

STRAWBERRIES & CREAM FROZEN
"Yogurt" Popsicles

INGREDIENTS:

- 1 cup heavy cream
- 1 cup sour cream
- ½ cup frozen strawberries
- 10 drops liquid vanilla stevia

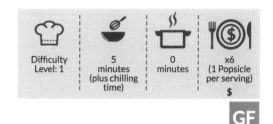

Difficulty Level: 1 | 5 minutes (plus chilling time) | 0 minutes | x6 (1 Popsicle per serving) $

GF

DIRECTIONS:

1. Add all ingredients to a high-speed blender, and blend until smooth.
2. Pour into 6 Popsicle molds and freeze for 4-6 hours or until completely hardened before serving.

Preparation Instructions:

Feel free to use any berries of choice in this recipe.

Serving Suggestions:

You can dunk the top of the Popsicles into melted unsweetened dark chocolate and set in the freezer for 10 minutes for an even more decadent treat.

Nutritional Information:

Carbs: 3g

Fiber: 0g

Net Carbs: 3g

Fat: 15g

Protein: 2g

Calories: 155

ORANGE *Creamsicles*

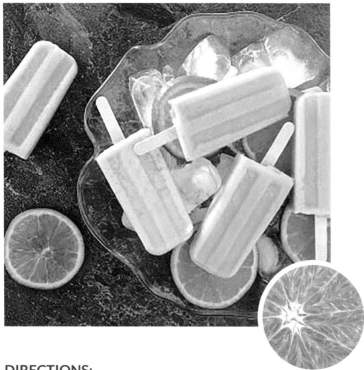

Difficulty Level: 1	5 minutes (plus chilling time)	0 minutes	x6 (1 popsicle per serving) $

INGREDIENTS:

- 1 cup heavy cream (use full-fat unsweetened coconut milk for a paleo version)
- ½ cup unsweetened almond milk
- ¼ cup freshly squeezed orange juice
- 10 drops liquid vanilla stevia

DIRECTIONS:

1. Add all ingredients to a high-speed blender, and blend until smooth.
2. Pour into 6 Popsicle molds and freeze for 4-6 hours or until completely hardened before serving.

Preparation Instructions:

You can use coconut milk in place of the heavy cream for a dairy-free version.

Serving Suggestions:

Drizzle the Popsicle with unsweetened chocolate syrup if desired.

Nutritional Information:

Carbs: 2g

Fiber: 0g

Net Carbs: 2g

Fat: 8g

Protein: 1g

Calories: 77

SAVORY MOCHA *Milkshake*

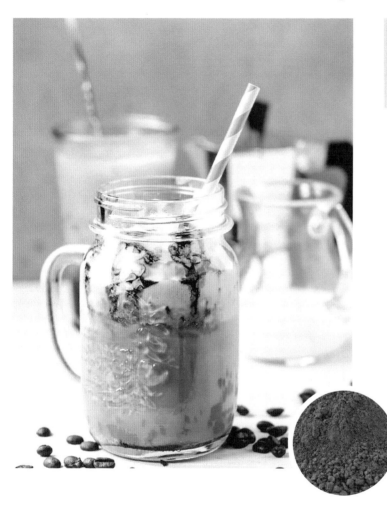

Difficulty Level: 1	5 minutes	0 minutes	x2 (approx. ½ cup per serving) $

GF

INGREDIENTS:

- 1 cup heavy cream
- 2 Tbsp. butter, melted
- ½ cup brewed coffee, chilled
- 1 Tbsp. unsweetened almond butter
- 1 Tbsp. raw cocoa nibs
- 1 handful of ice

- **Optional Toppings:** Whipped cream and no sugar added chocolate syrup

Preparation Instructions:

Use coconut milk in place of the heavy cream and eliminate the butter for a dairy-free version.

Serving Suggestions:

Serve with a dollop of unsweetened whipped cream.

DIRECTIONS:

1. Add all ingredients to a high-speed blender, and blend until smooth.
2. Pour into glasses and serve.
3. If using, top with whipped cream and no sugar added chocolate syrup.

Nutritional Information:

Carbs: 5g	**Fat:** 41g
Fiber: 1g	**Protein:** 3g
Net Carbs: 4g	**Calories:** 390

COCONUT CHOCOLATE
Chip Popsicles

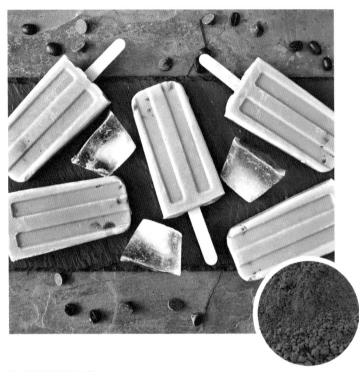

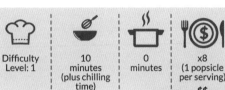

Difficulty Level: 1	10 minutes (plus chilling time)	0 minutes	x8 (1 popsicle per serving) $$

GF **DF** **P**

INGREDIENTS:

- 2 cups full-fat unsweetened coconut milk
- ½ cup coconut butter
- 1 tsp. pure vanilla extract
- ¼ cup chopped walnuts
- 10 drops liquid stevia
- 4 Tbsp. unsweetened dark chocolate chips

DIRECTIONS:

1. Add coconut milk, coconut butter, vanilla, walnuts, and stevia to a high-speed blender or food processor. Blend to combine.
2. Fold in the chocolate chips.
3. Pour into Popsicle molds and freeze for 4-6 hours or until completely solid before serving.

Preparation Instructions:

You can use any nut butter of choice in this recipe.

Serving Suggestions:

Drizzle the Popsicles with unsweetened chocolate syrup if desired.

Nutritional Information:

Carbs: 11g

Fiber: 6g

Net Carbs: 5g

Fat: 30g

Protein: 4g

Calories: 311

CHOCOLATE & ALMOND
Mint Pudding

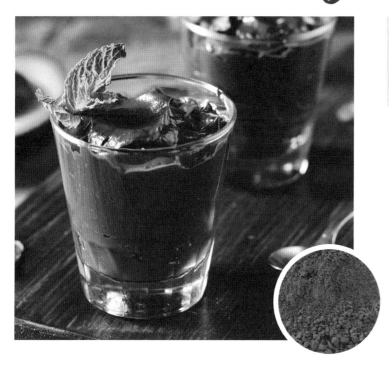

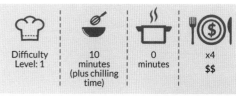

Difficulty Level: 1 | 10 minutes (plus chilling time) | 0 minutes | x4 $$

GF DF P

INGREDIENTS:

- 2 very ripe avocados, pitted and peeled
- ¼ cup full-fat unsweetened coconut milk
- ¼ cup raw unsweetened cocoa powder
- ½ tsp. almond extract
- ¼ tsp. pure peppermint extract
- 10 drops liquid stevia
- ⅛ tsp. sea salt

DIRECTIONS:

1. Add all the ingredients to a blender or food processor, and blend until creamy.
2. Chill for 30 minutes before enjoying.
3. Once chilled, enjoy right away.

Preparation Instructions:

You can use heavy cream in place of the coconut milk if not avoiding dairy.

Serving Suggestions:

Serve with chopped almonds if desired.

Nutritional Information:

Carbs: 13g

Fiber: 9g

Net Carbs: 4g

Fat: 24g

Protein: 3g

Calories: 253

HOMEMADE STRAWBERRY WHIPPED
Cream Parfait

INGREDIENTS:

- 1 cup heavy whipping cream
- 1 tsp. pure vanilla extract
- 10 drops of liquid vanilla stevia
- 1 cup strawberries, halved

Difficulty Level: 2 | 20 minutes | 0 minutes | x4 (approx. ¼ cup per serving) $$

DIRECTIONS:

1. Make whipped cream by adding the heavy whipping cream to a large bowl with the vanilla extract and stevia.
2. Whip using a handheld mixer until stiff peaks form.
3. Add half of the strawberries to the base of a glass jar or large bowl and top with half of the whipped cream.
4. Repeat these 2 layers.
5. Divide into 4 servings and serve.

Preparation Instructions:

You can use full-fat unsweetened coconut milk for a dairy-free version.

Serving Suggestions:

Serve with freshly chopped mint leaves for added flavor.

Nutritional Information:

Carbs: 4g

Fiber: 1g

Net Carbs: 3g

Fat: 11g

Protein: 1g

Calories: 118

Printed in Great Britain
by Amazon